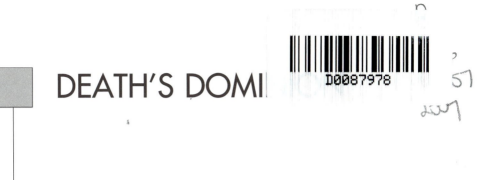

DEATH'S DOMI

FACING DEATH

Series editor: David Clark, Professor of Medical Sociology,
University of Lancaster

The subject of death in late modern culture has become a rich field of theoretical, clinical and policy interest. Widely regarded as a taboo until recent times, death now engages a growing interest among social scientists, practitioners and those responsible for the organization and delivery of human services. Indeed, how we die has become a powerful commentary on how we live, and the specialized care of dying people holds an important place within modern health and social care.

This series captures such developments. Among the contributors are leading experts in death studies, from sociology, anthropology, social psychology, ethics, nursing, medicine and pastoral care. A particular feature of the series is its attention to the developing field of palliative care, viewed from the perspectives of practitioners, planners and policy analysts; here several authors adopt a multidisciplinary approach, drawing on recent research, policy and organizational commentary, and reviews of evidence-based practice. Written in a clear, accessible style, the entire series will be essential reading for students of death, dying and bereavement, and for anyone with an involvement in palliative care research, service delivery or policy-making.

Current and forthcoming titles:

David Clark, Jo Hockley and Sam Ahmedzai (eds): *New Themes in Palliative Care*
David Clark and Jane E. Seymour: *Reflections on Palliative Care*
David Clark and Michael Wright: *Transitions in End of Life Care: Hospice and Related Developments in Eastern Europe and Central Asia*
Mark Cobb: *The Dying Soul: Spiritual Care at the End of Life*
Kirsten Costain Schou and Jenny Hewison: *Experiencing Cancer: Quality of Life in Treatment*
David Field, David Clark, Jessica Corner and Carol Davis (eds): *Researching Palliative Care*
Pam Firth, Gill Luff and David Oliviere: *Loss, Change and Bereavement in Palliative Care*
Anne Grinyer: *Cancer in Young Adults: Through Parents' Eyes*
Henk ten Have and David Clark (eds): *The Ethics of Palliative Care: European Perspectives*
Jenny Hockey, Jeanne Katz and Neil Small (eds): *Grief, Mourning and Death Ritual*
Jo Hockley and David Clark (eds): *Palliative Care for Older People in Care Homes*
David W. Kissane and Sidney Bloch: *Family Focused Grief Therapy*
Gordon Riches and Pam Dawson: *An Intimate Loneliness: Supporting Bereaved Parents and Siblings*
Lars Sandman: *A Good Death: On the Value of Death and Dying*
Jane E. Seymour: *Critical Moments: Death and Dying in Intensive Care*
Anne-Mei The: *Palliative Care and Communication: Experiences in the Clinic*
Tony Walter: *On Bereavement: The Culture of Grief*
Simon Woods: *Death's Dominion: Ethics at the End of Life*

DEATH'S DOMINION:
ETHICS AT THE END OF LIFE

SIMON WOODS

OPEN UNIVERSITY PRESS

Open University Press
McGraw-Hill Education
McGraw-Hill House
Shoppenhangers Road
Maidenhead
Berkshire
England
SL6 2QL

email: enquiries@openup.co.uk
world wide web: www.openup.co.uk

and Two Penn Plaza, New York, NY 10121–2289, USA

First published 2007

Copyright © Simon Woods, 2007

A catalogue record of this book is available from the British Library

ISBN 0 33521160 7 (pb) 0 335 21161 5 (hb)
ISBN 978 0335 21160 9 (pb) 978 0335 21161 6 (hb)

Library of Congress Cataloging-in-Publication Data
CIP data applied for

Typeset by YHT Ltd, London
Printed in UK by Bell & Bain Ltd, Glasgow

The *McGraw·Hill* Companies

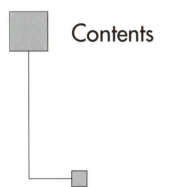

Contents

To Jane, Tom and Sarah.

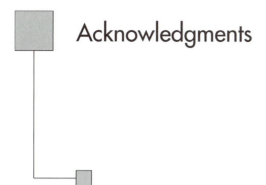

Acknowledgments

This book has been a long time in the writing and I am therefore particularly indebted to Rachael Gear of Open University Press for her patience, and especially grateful to David Clark for his encouragement, support, and critical comments. I am also indebted to those who know me as friend or colleague who have so frequently been drawn into discussion of the issues touched on in this book, but particular thanks go to Lars Sandman and Steve Edwards for their constructive criticism, to Tom Shakespeare for his lively debate of the issues, and to Anne Lepine who has her own unique perspective on these issues. I would also like to thank Kluwer Academic Press and Humana Press for permission to use sections of some previously published material and figures. Finally, it goes almost without saying, that the faults and weaknesses of the arguments and analysis I claim entirely for myself.

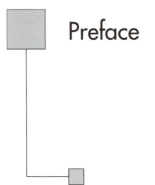

Preface

Within the Facing Death series we have done our best to give a prominent place to the works of moral philosophers and those engaged with bioethics. Among these we can list an edited collection entitled *The Ethics of Palliative Care*[i] as well as the work of Lars Sandman on *A Good* Death[ii]. In addition some related titles, such as *Reflections on Palliative Care*[iii] as well as the ethnographic studies we have published by Jane Seymour[iv] and Anne Mei[v]. They all engage at some point with ethical and moral issues surrounding modern end of life care in different settings.

I am therefore delighted to welcome to the series this new book by Simon Woods. He and I first met when we collaborated on a the European *Pallium* project that did so much to raise awareness about how the history and philosophy of palliative care are woven together with a range of values and beliefs that suffuse clinical practice in a variety of countries and cultures. I was impressed in that project by Simon's analytic reasoning and his ability to test to destruction' some cherished values within the world of palliative care. Whilst never hostile or mischievous, *Death's Dominion* does pose a number of questions that are extremely relevant to palliative care policy and practice and will be read with interest by anyone who has been following recent debates about palliative and end of life care and the ways in which they are evolving in the modern world. Simon Woods highlights the struggles that exist between a version of palliative care that remains rooted in Christian axiology and that which has embraced secular liberal ethics in the west. Germane to this is the rise of the concept of autonomy to the status of bioethical principle that is shaping all healthcare. There is justifiable scepticism at this approach and we are treated here to a fascinating counter-argument that is rooted in communitarian ethics. Nor does the book eschew specific clinical issues and there are useful chapters on the debates around end of life sedation as well as assisted dying and euthanasia. The conclusion leaves us with much on which to reflect concerning our rights and expectations for a good death'

This is a philosophical book written by one with experience at the clinical coalface. It is a worthy addition to the Facing Death series and adds significantly to wider debates about ethics and morals at the end of life. I commend it to all practitioners, ethicists and social scientists who are concerned with the unfolding moral landscape of hospice and palliative care.

David Clark

References

[i] Ten Have, H and Clark, D *The Ethics of Palliative Care: European Perspectives.* Buckingham: Open University Press, 2002.

[ii] Sandman, L *A Good Death: On the value of death and dying.* Maidenhead: Open University Press, 2005

[iii] Clark, D and Seymour, J (19999) *Reflections on Palliative Care.* Buckingham: Open University Press, vii-viii

[iv] Seymour, J.E. (2001) *Critical Moments: Death and Dying in Intensive Care.* Buckingham: Open University Press.

[v] The, A-M (2002) *Palliative Care and Communication: Experiences in the clinic.* Buckingham: Open University Press.

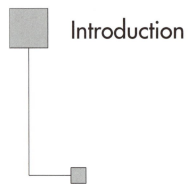

Introduction

This book has grown out of my long-standing interest in death, end-of-life decisions and palliative care. Working as a cancer nurse, I have witnessed many deaths some of which were 'good' and some of which were 'bad', some were brave, most were tragic and some were a peaceful release. However, these are my words and my evaluations. Although virtually all of the deaths from cancer that I witnessed were in a sense 'bad' because they were premature, and robbed the individual of the length and quality of life they had taken for granted would be theirs. The surviving friends and family had not only to witness the progress of the disease, but the dying, the death and then move on to live a life without their loved one.

As a nurse I found these experiences profound, often distressing, but sometimes also satisfying that we as nurses, doctors and other health workers had been able to help to ease the passing for both patient and family. I was therefore not only a witness, but actively involved as a professional attempting to achieve a good standard of care. It was from this perspective that I began to realize what good palliative care might be able to achieve.

I also had an intellectual interest in death and dying; as a philosophy graduate I was trained to think about the phenomenon that confronted us in our everyday experience. The fact of death is something that all philosophers find both disturbing and intriguing. Perhaps this is because philosophy is an activity of the mind and the realization that the stream of thoughts that accompany our waking moments might abruptly end is particularly alarming to a philosopher. As my philosophical studies also included ethics it was not merely the fact of death that was intriguing, but also the beliefs and the values they imply, which provoked reflection.

This book is about death, and the issues and ethical dilemmas faced at the end of life. The book begins by considering ethics more broadly, and explores the nature of moral significance and the different ethical perspectives taken on the value and sanctity of life. My own approach to ethics is rooted in pragmatism, a theory that I explain, then justify as appropriate to thinking about palliative care and end-of-life decisions.

In chapter 2 of this book, I consider the concept of the 'good death' within a philosophical framework based upon axiology. Axiology is the theory of value and, in this context, I explore the possible 'good-making' characteristics, or, parameters of the good death. I use a number of different thought experiments to explore and 'test' some intuitions about the good death, the natural death and the engineering of our dying. The philosopher Wittgenstein (1958) remarked that 'Death is not an event in life' — this is true, but the dying *is* an event for the dying person. Must we be forced to live through the dying merely for the sake of completion? Is death after palliative care a better or worse ending than a death deliberately and rationally precipitated by a person who wishes to control the means and timing of their end?

Chapter 3 turns specifically to palliative care and its underpinning values. Here, I trace the history of palliative care from its first beginnings in the early modern hospice movement. I argue that, although palliative care began within a Christian axiology, it has evolved to the point where it is possible to ask whether palliative care has maintained a distinct value set or whether it has become absorbed into the liberal secular ethics of western medicine? This chapter also explores the attempts by contemporary commentators and practitioners to conceptualize palliative care, describe its relationships to other branches of medicine and identify the ethical basis of its practises. My own analysis of palliative care values is that there has been an attempt to maintain a framework of values that is distinct from secular liberal ethics, but that the medicalization of palliative care has brought pressure on the palliative care community to adopt the secular liberal ethics of the west.

Chapters 4 and 5 explore the conceptual and practical implications of the palliative care axiology. In chapter 4, I concentrate on the concept of autonomy and its status in contemporary ethics. I first map out the liberal origins of this concept before offering a critique from the perspective of communitarianism. It is within a communitarian ethical framework, that I see the most likely philosophical home for palliative care values. In chapter 5 the communitarian model of palliative care values, developed in the previous chapter, is examined and an ethical framework as a practical application of the communitarian approach to autonomy is described.

Chapter 6 turns to an analysis of the meaning and role of sedation in terminal care. Efficient methods of achieving deep sedation mean it is possible to render a person insensible through their dying. The philosopher Torbjorn Tännsjö (2004) described deep sedation as 'terminal sedation' and suggested that this is something to offer as an alternative to euthanasia. However, can 'terminal sedation' be distinguished from forms of killing? Some argue that, even if it can, it would still contradict the goals of palliative care. The use of deep sedation raises some important questions. Is it nobler to suffer, rather than to bring about our own ending? Must a person experience their dying in order to have a good death? What, if anything, is the moral distinction between death after a period of insensible living and death at an earlier time? What sorts of distinctions help to clarify and justify the divide between the permissible and the illegitimate in this context, are actions always worse than omissions? In this chapter I argue, following Materstvedt and Kaasa (2000), for the adoption of 'palliative sedation' as an alternative to 'terminal sedation' and suggest the possible grounds for discriminating between different appropriate uses of this intervention.

Chapter 7 turns to the issue of killing and assisted dying. Here, I discuss some of the common arguments and distinctions that attempt to draw a clear line between what is part of palliative care and what is its antithesis. My argument here is that, because palliative care accepts the legitimacy of engineering some of the parameters of a good death, even where such interventions hasten death itself, then applying the criteria of appropriate and proportionate interventions, some forms of assisted dying are consistent with palliative care ethics and values.

My approach in this book will be philosophical. By this, I mean that I will employ philosophical methods and techniques to explore the questions posed. Some of the techniques will seem fantastical, but this is just the philosopher's way of testing ideas to the point of destruction and I hope that the purpose of such flights of fancy will be clear to the reader. Philosophical methods are, however, fundamentally about critique and argument, and to this end I will be subjecting some of the standard arguments and claims around end-of-life issues to philosophical analysis. I also hope that my arguments and analysis will encourage the reader to think about and explore these issues, both within their own thoughts and through the vehicle we have for sharing thought, through language and discussion. My approach, as I will explain, will be pragmatic and practical, and so at times my arguments will be in the more controlled tradition of applied ethics, because this is not a book solely for the armchair philosopher, but for those who work with death and dying.

This book, and others like it, need to be written, not because the issues and questions addressed are necessarily new, but because we can only benefit from continued opportunities to reflect on these important questions — these are questions that won't go away.

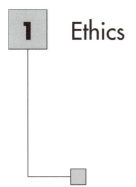

1 Ethics

Introduction

A single chapter can never do justice to what has taken volumes and centuries to consider. Nevertheless, I believe that it is necessary to set out the basic approach to ethics adopted in this book. My purpose in this chapter is to set out, as unambiguously as possible, the parameters of the ethical approach that drives the arguments in subsequent chapters. In doing so there is also a need to map out some of the established territory. Readers who are familiar with this ground may choose to move on, although I would suggest that what I discuss in this chapter is relevant to understanding the more substantive arguments that follow.

The principal concerns of this book are the ethics of end-of-life decisions, but it is, of course, nonsense to talk only of the *end* of life as if this were a peculiar episode, which can be considered in isolation from the rest of one's life. Therefore, in this chapter I begin with a brief outline of what ethics is, beginning with the concept of moral value or, as I prefer, moral *significance*. I then turn to the concept of the sanctity of life, exploring the traditional and contemporary critical views of this concept. The traditional view of the sanctity of life is pertinent to end-of-life decisions, since the fact of being alive is argued by some to bestow inviolable moral significance on the person in a way that places absolute constraints upon ethics at the end of life. By contrast, the principle of respect for autonomy has grown to a similar status amongst its advocates. Both values are sincerely held by many and regarded as moral cornerstones; however, I shall argue that to cling to such absolutes without evaluating how such beliefs cohere with other values is to ultimately undermine ethics.

Any consideration of ethics must turn to a discussion of the concept of the person and the theories of *personhood* as they are prosaically described in the philosophical literature. This concept is important since there has been a move by some to draw a distinction between life and morally significant life, and between being human and being a person. An account of this concept is necessary because being a person, that is, having the qualities that bestow personhood, has become the most important rival to the traditional view that being *human* is the ground of moral value. Personhood can therefore be seen as challenging what might be regarded as the more traditional beliefs about what kind of entity has moral value. From the consideration of personhood, I turn to the concept of autonomy, and how a particular understanding of this concept can inform moral choices and decisions at the end of life. I conclude the chapter with a defence of the anthropomorphic person and an account of the pragmatic approach to ethics that I shall be employing throughout the book.

Ethics and moral significance

Ethics concerns our notions of good and bad, right and wrong. However, in relation to what? The application of these concepts requires a prior understanding of *moral significance*, which is the grounds for distinguishing the sort of 'thing' or entity that has moral significance. We seem to have some basic intuitions that inform our beliefs on this matter; for example, there seems to be an obvious difference between kicking a stone and kicking a cat. This is where, in discussing ethics, things become complicated very quickly. For example, let us presume that the only harm done in kicking a stone is potentially to the kicker's toe, since the very idea of whether a thing can be harmed or not is related to the capacity that thing has to feel pain. A stone, being inanimate or non-sentient, is not the sort of thing that can be hurt, but what of a cat? Presuming that the kick causes the cat pain then is the cat hurt? This seems to be obviously the case, since if a thing can feel pain then it can be hurt, since pain and hurt are of the same category. However, to ask whether the cat is wronged by the kick is to introduce a very different category — a moral category. To answer this question seems to require consideration of at least two further issues: is the cat the sort of entity that can be wronged and is the kicker the sort of thing that can do wrong? Our judgement regarding the cat's status will rest on some account of its capacity to both *feel* pain and to *be* wronged. Our evaluation of the kick will rest on the capacity of the kicker not just to inflict pain, but to *do* wrong. A quick, if crude, thought experiment throws the issue into relief: imagine a world populated by a limited number of species, cows, cats, dogs and rats, and presume that this means no people. Imagine these animals doing what animals do, cows kicking dogs, dogs chasing cats, cats catching rats. The question is does it make sense to ask whether the cow, in kicking out, both hurts and wrongs the dog? Does the cat in catching the rat both kill it and murder it? I would suggest that this imaginary world contains pains and hurts, but not wrongs, killings and deaths, but not murders. I accept that there might be a debate as to whether some non-human animals, chimpanzees or dolphins, for example, might be capable of being wronged and doing wrong. Some philosophers, such as Peter Singer (1994) and Alasdair MacIntyre (1999), seriously address this issue, but I will only touch on the matter here.

So a further idea relevant to understanding ethics is the possibility of distinguishing between things that have moral significance and things that have the capacity for moral agency. Bonnie Steinbock makes the following observation:

> Beings that have moral status must be capable of caring about what is done to them. They must be capable of being made, if only in a rudimentary sense, happy or miserable, comfortable or distressed. Whatever reasons we may have for preserving or protecting non-sentient beings, these reasons do not refer to their own interests. For without conscious awareness, beings cannot have interests. Without interests they cannot have a welfare of their own. Without a welfare of their own, nothing can be done for their sake. Hence they lack moral Standing or status.
>
> (Steinbock 1992:5)

Steinbock's account is clearly only helpful to a degree. While it gives us grounds for recognizing that both human and non-human animals have moral significance, in so far as they have interests, it omits a second crucial part of the equation, which must be completed if we are to have an account of where ethics begins. A thing can only have moral status if there exists an agent capable of taking those interests into account. In other words, there must exist a being capable of giving reasons for or of being held accountable for its actions, in order for there to be moral agency. It is only when there is a being capable of giving reasons, of justifying its actions, can there be any talk of ethics. Without such beings there can only be pleasure or pain, but there cannot be any right or wrong.

A necessary condition for ethics and, hence, for morality of any kind, is that there are beings with the capacity for agency of a particular kind; that is, they must be capable of forming reasons as a cause of their actions. While I readily accept that there is at least a theoretical possibility that non-human animals may posses such a capacity, I believe that most will agree that it is human beings who are the paradigm example of the sort of thing that has such a capacity. To summarize, ethics is only possible if there are both entities with interests *and* entities with the capacity for moral agency. Moral agency is a necessary condition for ethics, since moral agency implies that reasons can be the cause of actions and ethics is centrally concerned with the adequacy of the reasons that justify action.

Ethics is therefore only possible if there is an entity with the capacity for giving reasons for its actions. Of course, having such a capacity is no guarantee that a person will act ethically or morally; in this book I do not distinguish between the terms. To act ethically is to use this capacity to justify one's action in terms of right and wrong. More formally, this involves the making of moral arguments, but also the critical scrutiny of the reasons given in such arguments for what is argued for, for the basis of what is right or wrong. What is judged to be right or wrong must be defended by reasons, and the adequacy of reasons can always be challenged. The capacity for moral agency is, of course, related to the concept of moral significance, so I return to the account of moral significance.

The next step in the argument is to ask whether any distinctions can be drawn between the moral significance of those entities that have interests? One line of argument takes the view that there is equality among the entities that have interests. In other words, equal weight ought to be given to the interests of different entities. This is a theory sometimes referred to as *species egalitarianism* and amounts to the claim that all life is of equal moral worth. On this view, our restricted world of cows, dogs, cats and rats, since it is a world in which such creatures can have their interests furthered or thwarted, would count as a world of moral significance, that is; a world containing morally significant beings. However, this is not what we mean when we talk of ethics, and of right and wrong. The intuitive distinctions we draw between killing cholera, cooking a carrot, kicking a cat and harming a human being, indicates one of the obvious challenges such a theory faces. I therefore do not intend dwelling on this theory further. A more discerning argument is made by Peter Singer (1995), who argues that we ought to give moral weight to the interests of living things, but that we are justified in giving different weight to different individuals, even within a species, according to the particular characteristics of the individual. Singer is against the idea that we can justifiably generalize about the moral significance of a thing based merely upon species. It is from this position that he argues that even human life may differ in its moral value. However, even Singer's argument can only get off the ground if there exists at least some entities capable of forming moral judgements.

The idea that there may be important differences among the class of things that have moral significance seems a particularly important claim in the context of ethics. Establishing the grounds of such a distinction is necessary if such differences are to feature as components of moral claims and argument. There is a common intuition that there is a moral hierarchy, in which it is assumed that humans are at the top having superiority over other living creatures. The biblical view, as expressed in the book of Genesis, that God gave Man dominion over all the animals is but one account in which Man's moral status is established by divine fiat. John Harris (1985) pursues this same intuition, but without the presumption that any such distinction is divinely decreed. Harris asks:

When we ask what makes human life valuable we are trying to identify those features, whatever they are, which both incline us and entitle us to value ourselves and one another, and which license our belief that we are more valuable (and not just to ourselves) than animals, or fish or plants. We are looking for the basis of the belief that it is morally right to choose to save the life of a person rather than that of a dog where both cannot be saved, and our belief that this is not merely a form of prejudice in the favour of our own species but is capable of justification.

(Harris 1985: 10)

This quotation from Harris reveals that he is sceptical or at least agnostic as to the specifically moral significance of species. Implicit in Harris's argument is the claim that if the decision to save the person over the dog is a specifically moral claim, then there must be specifically moral reasons why this is so, and not merely a blind preference for one of our own species or alternatively for a furry companion of another. However, an important traditional way in which this distinction has been made has been to assert this very point that the highest moral status is exclusively reserved for members of the human race. The language of religion is often used to express this claim so that the moral significance of humans is talked of in terms of the *sacredness* or sanctity of human life. If something has sanctity, then its status is of the highest order of value, of infinite value. The traditional account of the sanctity of life argument makes the quite specific claim that it is *all* and *only* human life that has such value. To begin with, I shall concentrate on this claim. This said, the mere possibility that other non-human forms of life may have a moral status, which equals that of humans, is an important consideration for reasons that will become clear as we continue.

There are, of course, both theological and secular versions of the sanctity of life argument, but what I call the 'traditional' form of the argument is theological, informed by such religious beliefs that humans are made in God's image or that humans are uniquely in possession of a soul. This form of the sanctity of human life is prevalent in Islamic, Judaeo-Christian and other religious traditions. The Judaeo-Christian influence on Western thought has been a profound one, forming the bedrock of the moral and the legal conceptions behind, for example, the prohibition on taking innocent human life. This is, of course, a gross simplification of some important ideas and as with any simplification there is a danger that injustice is done to such ideas. What such ideas have in common is a broad agreement that the source of the moral significance of human life is transcendental; that is, its source is outside of human life coming from God, rather than human life itself.

There is also an important and related theory, deriving from the Greek philosopher Aristotle (1925), which should be mentioned here for completeness. Although Aristotle's influence has been a profound one, strongly associated with the traditional theological approaches and perhaps most closely with Roman Catholic traditions, it does differ in one significant way. The Aristotelian account of the value of an individual does not, in principle, rely upon the existence of a God, offering, not a theological account, but rather an objective *teleological* account. David Oderberg (2000a, b) gives an interpretation of what he calls 'the traditional approach' without any overt reference to a God or religion. This point is relevant because those who adopt a critical view of the sanctity of life doctrine often object on the basis that it is wrong to expect non-believers to live their lives according to the creed of believers. Those who object to euthanasia or assisted suicide, for example, often do so on specifically religious grounds. An argument for the sanctity of life that is a-religious would be a stronger argument against those that support euthanasia, but have no religious beliefs.

What is a teleological account? The term is derived from the Greek word *telos* meaning end or goal, and Oderberg quotes approvingly from Aristotle:

> Every art and every enquiry, and similarly every action and pursuit, is thought to aim at some good; and for this reason the good has rightly been declared to be that at which all things aim.
> (Aristotle 1925: Nicomachean Ethics 1094a)

With this Aristotelian conception in mind, Oderberg goes on to unpack what he sees as the most fundamental ethical concept; the concept of 'good' (Oderberg 2000a). Oderberg develops the argument in a way that echoes what I have already explored in terms of moral significance. Oderberg puts the point in the following way. It makes sense only of certain categories of thing, living things, to say that things go well or badly for them. With regard to all manner of living things we can readily think of the conditions that enable the thing to flourish, or else struggle and perish. This is true of a host of living things from plants to bacteria to people. The more complex the animal then the more complex the conditions required in order that the animal may flourish. The most complex of animals is, of course, the human being, whose complexity is not simply a matter of degree, but of order, since the human being possesses rationality and in virtue of this:

> ... he is capable of *reasoning about how he should live his life*. He spends much of his time *ordering* things so that he lives a certain kind of life. He *reflects* on how he wants to live and *proposes* certain things to himself as worthy or as not worthy. Whether it be in the area of work, social life, family, health, mental or physical pursuits, from the moment he is *capable* of thinking about his life he *does* so think, and

therefore thinks about how he should arrange those ingredients that go to make up what he believes will be a *good life* for him. (sic.)

(Oderberg 2000a: 36; original emphasis)

It is important to spend a little time in spelling out the implications of the Aristotelian view for the traditional position as it has implications for many of the issues to be discussed in this book. When Oderberg talks of the 'good life' for man he means that the *telos* or end for mankind is to live the 'good life' — the sort of life in which man can flourish. Of course, there are many different kinds of 'good' and the general term does not immediately distinguish between the good of eating and drinking well, of exercise, of friendship, of learning and thinking, and what are the more obviously moral goods of right conduct, doing the right thing. What this general Aristotelian account does acknowledge is that there are many different kinds of 'good' and that these are interrelated, nested within one another, each contributing to the overall good life for mankind. Most people enjoy eating and drinking, and dining out is a great source of pleasure, not just for the enjoyment of flavours and textures in the food and drink, but for the occasion itself, the company and so on. However, although each of these features may be a good end in itself they are not the most important ends in life. Many people will identify with the dining out experience that has become an episode of overindulgence and thereby self-defeating of the goal aimed at. According to the Aristotelian view, to understand the *true* end of eating and drinking well, we must think about how eating and drinking contribute to nutrition, which is necessary for healthy functioning of the human species. The good life for man is necessarily complex given man's range of needs and capacities. The good life involves living well across a range of goods, nutrition and health, relationships, civic responsibilities and, of course, exercising rationality both for it's own sake, and as necessary to the process of pursuing the goals of other activities and pursuits. An example given by Oderberg is that of playing the piano. To play the piano, he argues, is to play the piano *well*. This does not mean that unless you are a virtuoso musician you may as well not bother, because of course, how would anyone ever start to play the piano? Playing the piano, he argues can be distinguished from merely tinkering with the keys, placing the cat upon the keyboard because the sound amuses you or pounding the keys with your fists as a release of tension. What playing the piano means is that there is a goal to playing the piano that can be described as 'playing the piano well'.

The point is that the art itself, and every serious attempt to practise it, has good execution as its intrinsic objective ... everything that a person does, *everything*, aims at something deemed good or worthwhile.

(Oderberg 2000a: 37)

To play the piano, therefore, is to aim at this end, with implications for how one acts, developing the necessary skills through conscientious practice, devoting serious time to study, seeking tuition from an appropriate teacher and so on. This model, Oderberg argues, is true for all aspects of living well and the multiple talents required for living well are described as the *virtues*.

The good that something aims at is described, according to this Aristotelian view, as the *intrinsic* good. However, activities and pursuits may be given *extrinsic* goods as their goal, that is, purposes that serve our own ends, merely deemed 'good' by the individual because they are instrumental to some desired goal. Playing a Chopin piece with more fortissimo than necessary because you take delight in annoying your neighbour may suit your purpose, but is inconsistent with playing the piano well and, come to think of it, it is inconsistent with being a good neighbour. Your own goal of annoying your neighbour is merely an instrumental good not to be confused with the intrinsic good of playing the piano.

This digression into the Aristotelian influence on ethics is useful because not only does it raise the possibility that there is a good life for mankind, but that humans must also use their intellect and rationality to pursue an understanding of what it is to live such a life. We shall return to a consideration of these issues in chapter 2 when I discuss the good death, and also in chapters 4 and 5 when I consider the principle of respect for autonomy in the context of palliative care.

The account of the 'good' may seem obvious enough, even if the concept of the good life for man, given this very brief introduction, seems plausible if rather abstract. However, what is apparent is that a pattern emerges, that there is some agreement, even from the diverse approaches different people may take, that to engage in ethics is to engage in a dispute over different conceptions of what is good. However, the point of this section is not merely to show that there is some broad agreement about what it is to engage in ethics. The real purpose here is to show that the Aristotelian approach, like the specifically theistic accounts, presumes that there is an intrinsic moral value, which attaches to the fact that an entity is a live human being. It is no coincidence that some latter-day Aristotelians also believe that life is a gift from God, but this does not diminish from the altogether independent claim that life is an intrinsic good. Oderberg makes the point in this way:

> The good of life then is fundamental in a way that other goods are not. Two individuals could live equally flourishing lives even though for one it is, say, art that is the most important thing, and for the other, knowledge. But life itself cannot be similarly demoted in favour of other goods. The good of life is part of the very moral framework within which the evaluation of action can take place, because every action is evaluated in terms of its contribution to a *good life*. No

person can flourish without being alive in the first place, so if he deliberately undercuts his life in pursuit of other goods, he will soon have no goods to pursue whatsoever.

(Oderberg 2000a: 142–3)

So for both theistic and non-theistic approaches the essential good is life itself, this is not to say that being alive is not, in a sense, instrumental to living a good life; of course it is, because unless you are alive there can be no goods to achieve. Supporters of the life-as-a-fundamental-good also claim that because life is good in and of itself, then a number of further truths follow:

- Life is an intrinsic good independent of whether X is aware that they are alive.
- Life is an intrinsic good independent of whether X, being aware, *believes* that their life is such a good.

The argument that life is an intrinsic good therefore has obvious implications for ethics at the end of life. The first proposition has implications for cases like those of Anthony Bland (Singer 1994) and Maria Schiavo (Gostin 2005), and the many other cases of individuals left in a persistent vegetative state, alive, but unaware. The second proposition has implications for cases like those of Diane Pretty and Ms B both of whom were alive and fully aware of their situation. Diane Pretty, who in the advanced stages of Multiple Sclerosis, went to the Court of Appeal in an attempt to achieve lawful recognition of her right to assisted suicide. Ms B, a paralysed woman dependent on a ventilator, needed to take similar steps in order for her right to refuse life-sustaining treatment to be recognized (Boyd 2002). What will be clear to any reader familiar with palliative care is the resonance of these themes with the ethical position adopted by the advocates and supporters of palliative care. Evidence given to the House of Lords by the Association of Palliative Medicine (APM1993) affirmed the importance of respect for patient autonomy, but also that: 'The doctor should show respect for life and acceptance of death by understanding that: treatment should never have the induction of death as its specific aim' (1993: 2) and 'without any degree of religious conviction, it is justifiable to assert that life has value and meaning. Euthanasia poses the risk that an opportunity for growth will be lost and that life will be devalued' (1993: 4).

More recently, the House of Lords Select Committee on the Assisted Dying for the Terminally Ill (ADTI) Bill (2005a, b) also heard evidence from members and supporters of the palliative care community. In his statement to the Committee, John Finnis said:

At present there is a clear principle: never intend to kill the patient; never try to help patients to intentionally kill themselves. That is the Law, it is the long-established common morality, it is the ethic of the health care professions ... There is a 'bright' line, and though like other laws and principles it is not invariably respected it is not the least artificial or brittle; it rests on a rational principle that a person's life is the very reality of the person, and whatever your feelings of compassion you cannot intentionally try precisely to eliminate the persons reality and existence without disrespect to the person and their basic equality of worth with others.

(House of Lords Select Committee ADTI Bill 2005b: 553)

So, from the outset, it is therefore possible to establish that the ethical stance of palliative care is in line with a traditional morality and this position, along with relevant cases and issues, will be discussed in the body of this book.

The traditional view claims that the moral significance of a human life is therefore independent of any of the qualities of the individual life. The logical implication of this position is that all human life has the same moral significance, regardless of whether it is in the form of a foetus, a conscious, but terminally ill adult or permanently comatose individual. Once all of the implications of such a moral foundation are understood, then it follows that the necessity, the possibility even, of moral debate regarding some seemingly obvious moral dilemmas is removed. Adopting this view might plausibly be seen to evaporate many contemporary ethical problems, such as the right or wrong of destructive research on human embryos, deliberate termination of pregnancy, euthanasia and assisted suicide, because certain acts are deemed to be intrinsically wrong, wrong *in and of themselves*. If being human conveys an absolute moral status, as captured in the notion of what is sacred, there can be no justification for the taking of life that is sacred and, hence, there can be no further debate on such questions.

A parallel and now familiar account of the traditional sanctity of human life argument is conducted in terms of human rights. 'Rights' talk had its origins in the eighteenth century emerging from the rhetoric that accompanied the various rebellious upheavals and revolutions of that period. One of the most famous statements of rights *The Declaration of Independence of the Thirteen Colonies* July 4 1776 states:

We hold these truths to be self-evident, that all men are created equal, that they are endowed by their Creator with certain unalienable Rights, that among these are Life, Liberty and the pursuit of Happiness.

Although *The Declaration* suggests that the origins of such rights are the gift of a Creator, later rights talk sees rights as an intrinsic and inalienable aspect of being human. The European convention on Human Rights and its incorporation into English Law through the Human Rights Act 1998 (HRA) is an affirmation that to be human is to be a bearer of rights. The most fundamental of these is expressed in the Article 2 statement of the Right to Life (HRA 1998). An important difference between the theological and the rights-based versions of the sanctity of life argument is that the latter takes a different approach when drawing the boundaries to what may be legitimately disputed. The rights approach is more permissive in allowing for the possibility of deliberation when conflicts arise, although this does not necessarily imply consistency in approach. Such a conflict formed the basis of the debate and legal challenge over the legitimacy of abortion in the United States in the infamous case of *Roe v Wade* 1973 (Dworkin 1993). In this case, the liberty of the mother to decide what to do with her own body was given priority over the right to life of the foetus she was carrying. This decision was at odds with the traditional accounts of the sanctity of life and advocates of this tradition have continued to challenge the decision to this day. Inconsistencies can be observed between different states that, nevertheless, subscribe to human rights. Members of the European Union regard capital punishment as incompatible with human rights, whereas the United States regards this as compatible with their own constitution. Different countries within Europe and different States within the United States take quite different views on euthanasia and assisted dying, which suggests that the 'rights' base for the sanctity of life offers a scope for debate that the theological base of the traditional position does not. Which of these, therefore, is the basis of the contemporary palliative care position?

It is the traditional theological account of the sanctity of life I have in mind as I continue this discussion. Although there may be differences in detail in how sanctity of life arguments are made, whatever the detail, these accounts are attempts to distinguish the moral order to be applied to different kinds of life. A common ground among these traditional approaches is that it is not being alive that bestows moral worth, but rather uniquely human life that does so. These sorts of considerations feed into an account of the sanctity of life that can be given a standard format, which I shall refer to as the Sanctity of Life Doctrine — there is a common core of beliefs associated with this doctrine:

- that (human) life is of infinite value;
- that (human) life is of irreducible value;
- that (human) life is of equal value.

There are a number of implications of these three core beliefs that are relevant to this book because these beliefs can be seen to underpin palliative care philosophy. The first, that life is of infinite value, has been taken to imply that since infinity is indivisible then every part of life is of equal value. Such arguments are frequently used to generate the idea that life is valuable from the point at which it starts, which for some is conception, to the point at which it ends in death, with every moment between those points being of equal value. The implication of this view is that any deliberate foreshortening of life is wrong against something that has infinite value. Therefore, abortion at one point and euthanasia at another with suicide or murder occurring at any point in the interim being equal and grave wrongs. Again, what is distinctive about the traditional approach is the view that certain acts are wrong in and of themselves.

Re-valuing life

Moral philosophy since Aristotle has continued to explore the many different ways of characterizing the human good. One of the theories that have been most influential on contemporary ethics has been that developed by the modern philosophers of liberalism, most notably the founders of Utilitarianism, Jeremy Bentham (1789), and John Stuart Mill (1859). Bentham and Mill agreed that human experience was the key to understanding the human good, and that the relevant aspect of human experience is the propensity for feeling pleasure and pain. Since they believed that pleasure and pain could be quantified, they argued that what we ought to do, what is *right* in moral terms, is to commit ourselves to acting in ways likely to produce the greatest amount of pleasure (or happiness) over pain. Utilitarianism is the theory that the right thing to do is to maximize *utility* and minimize *disutility,* or, simplistically, maximize pleasure and avoid pain. Utilitarianism is perhaps the most well known of a group of theories known as consequentialism. Consequentialism holds that the moral rightness of an act depends entirely on whether the consequences of an act are better or worse than for an alternative act. According to consequentialism, in contrast to the traditional approach, no act is right or wrong in and of itself, but only in so far as it has good or bad consequences. This basic tenet of consequentialism is the subject of volumes of debate and, although we will return to some of these issues during the course of this book, I will for the moment consider just some of the implications of consequentialism for the present discussion.

There has been a move in contemporary ethics, of which utilitarianism has been the most important influence, to challenge the traditional basis for the moral significance of human beings. This seems to follow quite obviously, since if it is true that what matters morally is utility, and utility concerns the capacity to experience pleasure or pain, then clearly all kinds of animals other than humans, share this capacity. This takes us back to the point at which we began this chapter where we began to consider two questions, the nature of moral significance and how ethics gets started. On the first question, I argued that for anything to have moral significance it must be capable of having interests. The emphasis given to the capacity for experiencing pleasure and pain by utilitarianism identifies the most rudimentary basis for something's having interests. Although having interests may be a necessary condition for a thing to have moral status, this fact is not alone sufficient, since there must be something capable of weighing such interests in deciding the right course of action. Utilitarianism, in common with all moral theories regards human beings as having moral significance. Where the contemporary descendants of utilitarianism differ from traditional approaches to ethics, is in the view that it is only in virtue of the mental capacities human beings typically possess that they have moral significance. Philosophers such as Glover (1984), Harris (1985), Parfit (1991) and Singer (1995), to name but a few, have argued that the moral significance of human beings is misplaced in the traditional account and that a better account, that is, an account that offers a superior set of moral discriminations, is one that sees moral significance not as exclusive to human beings. It would be misleading to say that the traditional standpoint dismisses non-human animals as entirely lacking in interests that merit moral consideration, but rather traditional approaches to ethics regard being human as both necessary and sufficient for moral significance by fiat of divine decree. Those who are critical of this account, including the advocates of consequentialism, argue for an alternative account, which they consider is better able to draw moral differences both between human beings and other species, and also between different human beings. These contemporary views are attempts to describe the class of things of the highest moral status in such a way that it is not synonymous with being human. In addition, advocates of this approach claim to offer a way of enriching our capacity for making moral judgements by refining our ability to discriminate between competing moral claims. One of the ways in which the distinction between being human and having moral significance is drawn is by introducing a new category of the *person*.

Persons and moral significance

The first point to make in this discussion is that the term *person* is being used in a technical sense, rather than in its ordinary sense. Although this may seem confusing, the term is used in this way to illustrate that what endows a thing with moral significance of the highest order is in principle separable from other defining features such as species. So, for example, it is not for the fact that a human being is a member of the species *homo sapien* that they have moral significance, but rather in virtue of certain other capacities. On this view, for an entity to have moral significance, it must have at least the capacity to take an interest in its own welfare, but further, for talk of ethics to be meaningful, it must also be capable of acting on the basis of reasons, rather than mere instinct. The point of this argument is to show that the things with the greatest moral significance are those with both 'welfare' to care about and the capacity for acting on the basis of reasons. To have such a capacity requires a degree of intelligence and self-awareness of the kind that is usually unquestionably ascribed to adult human beings, which does not rule out the possibility that other, non-human beings may have such capacities and, hence, moral significance to the same degree. For some people, this may seem deeply counter-intuitive, after all is it not plainly obvious that a human being is *the* quintessential moral agent? This is precisely the point assumed by the traditional approach to ethics and is, indeed, shared to an extent by some of its critics. The traditional approach, however, assumes that the moral significance of a human being follows from the fact of their humanity. Whereas for those who take the *persons* approach, the moral significance of human beings is not in virtue of their being human, but rather that humans are the sort of entity that can possess the qualities that endow a thing with moral significance. What this means is that not only do humans have interests, but that they are capable of recognizing their own and other's interests, and of acting on the basis of reasons. However, on the person's view, it does not follow that because some human beings have moral significance that all humans do.

There are therefore important differences and similarities between the traditional and the *persons* view. The main difference between the two is that, in the traditional view, all and only human beings have moral significance as opposed to the view that only *persons* do. However, both viewpoints accept that whatever has such a moral status then all such things are moral equals, that is; they are all owed equal care, concern and consideration. Advocates of the *persons* approach cite the philosopher John Locke's definition of person, as an important influence upon contemporary accounts of the concept:

> ... to find wherein personal identity consists, we must consider what person stands for; which, I think, is a thinking intelligent Being, that has reason and reflection, and can consider it self as it self, the same thinking thing in different times and places'
>
> (Locke 1976 Bk. 2. xxvii: 162)

Locke's definition of the person renders most human beings *prima facie* examples of persons, but there are in principle at least two possible groups of exceptions. First, the possibility of non-human persons, since Locke's criteria are species non-specific. The as-yet-to-be proven existence of extra-terrestrials, may, in the event, prove to be both alien creatures and alien persons. More likely, perhaps, is the possibility of terrestrial non-human persons, with certain species of primate and sea mammal frequently put forward as the strongest candidates (Harris 1985; Singer 1995; MacIntyre 1999). Perhaps the most alarming implication of taking Locke's emphasis on these psychological characteristics as necessary for moral significance is that it allows the possibility of an entirely disembodied *person*. This conjures up a futuristic and, perhaps to some, a nightmarish image of some complex computer program being regarded as a person. This possibility is too distracting from the central concerns of this book; however, the science-fiction does serve a purpose in that it forces us to test, to the point of destruction, the idea that moral significance follows from the fact that one has the right kind of mental 'properties'. Whether we could extend the category of moral significance to include other species or even beings of a radically different kind is a separate question from whether we ought to. What concerns us here is the converse case, whether the category of *persons* can be contracted, to exclude some human beings from this category? This brings me to the second exception implied by Locke's criteria for person-hood, the possibility of human *non-persons*. According to the *persons* approach, being human is neither necessary nor sufficient for being a *person*. This seems quite plausible if we consider that a human corpse is still *human,* but it is no longer a *person*, the fact that it is now possible to culture human cells presents us with something that is both human and alive, but arguably not deserving of the equal concern and protection accorded to a person. There is, of course, a more troubling class of a human individual that is alive, but on the *persons* view is judged to be a non-*person* and, therefore, does not merit the equal concern and protection accorded to *persons*. As discussed, examples include the human foetus and those who are *irreversibly* unconscious or who permanently lack, through some other cause, the mental capacities deemed necessary for personhood. Advocates of the *persons* approach subscribe to two basic tenets, the first is that moral significance can differ in degree, and second, that being a live human being is not enough to endow an individual with the full moral status accorded to *persons*. This, it is argued, is in keeping with many of the practises common to human conduct that afford priority to the interests of the mother over the foetus, to the interests of the recipient of an organ donation over those of the 'beating-heart' donor and in many other trade-off situations. Thus, the observation that an individual is not a person becomes a key reason in arguments for the permissibility of abortion, and with greater relevance to end-of-life ethics, the withholding or withdrawing of treatment from indi-viduals who are permanently unconscious. The *persons* approach, if accepted, offers a logical approach to decision-making in these challenging circumstances. However, the *persons* approach does also seem deeply counter-intuitive to some other features of human valuing and attachment.

The traditional approach to ethics, which takes the view that being a live human individual is sufficient to convey the highest moral status, requires a process of reasoning which may also seem counter-intuitive. A problem common to both the traditional and the *persons* approach is that they appear to rule out from the ethical debate, albeit for contrary reasons, many issues that lie at the heart of what we see as fundamentally moral dilemmas and problems.

Saving the anthropocentric person

In this chapter I have been considering the question 'What matters morally'? In a book on ethics at the end of life, this does seem to be *the* pre-eminent question for all of us, when deciding the rights and wrongs of the many moral dilemmas that we face at the end of life. Most philosophical approaches are unashamedly foundationalist; seeking to find the ground, the first premise, on which the edifice can be constructed. In this chapter, we have consider the approach of traditional morality, but briefly also that of contemporary 'consequentialist' philosophers. Before developing my own approach, I will offer a critique of what I see as the inadequacies of the *person* approach and, in particular, how this approach has been developed by John Harris (1985; see also Woods 2006). Harris uses the concept of the *person* in the following way:

> In identifying the things that make human life valuable we will be pointing to the features that would make the existence of any being who possessed them valuable. It is important to have a word for such beings which is not simply anthropocentric or species-specific. I shall use the term *person* to stand for any being who has what it takes to be valuable in the sense described, whatever they are otherwise like.
>
> (Harris 1985: 9)

This passage is one example of where Harris acknowledges that the term *person* has a technical meaning that should be substituted by the reader for the established usage of this term, which loosely regards 'person' as synonymous with 'human being'. I disagree with Harris because, although he may claim more precision in this semantic shift, the common use of 'person', the anthropocentric person, is good enough as it stands, as messy and ambiguous as it may be. Harris's concept of the *person* raises a number of serious problems and here I shall address the following: that Harris's account of the *person* claims more precision in ethics than the subject is capable of. If we were to accept Harris's position then we would have to be prepared to relinquish issues that at the moment are deeply morally contentious and, in doing so, have to accept moral verdicts too far out of line with everyday moral intuitions. More broadly, Harris's approach oversimplifies the nature of human valuing and, hence, underestimates the role of human attachment in the context of ethics.

I have already outlined that the starting point for any moral theory is to delineate those things that have moral significance or, to use Harris's term, those things that have *value,* from those that do not. Without this basic discrimination ethics would be impossible. We need also to distinguish between things that deserve our moral concern from things that do not and crucially, to distinguish between things that can be imputed with moral responsibility and those that cannot. We can proceed in these tasks at a fairly intuitive level and without the need for too much philosophical sophistication, and my opening example of stones and cats was designed to make this point.

The basic argument is that the very idea of harming is related to the capacity a thing has to experience. So we may accept that an experiencing thing can be harmed, but to establish whether that same thing can be wronged requires two further considerations. Since 'wronging' is a moral category, we need to be satisfied on two counts, that something can *be* wronged and that something can *do* wrong.

Therefore, a necessary condition for ethics and, hence, for morality of any kind is that there are beings with the capacity for agency of a particular kind; that is, they must be capable of forming reasons as a cause of their actions. It seems reasonable to claim that the highest moral status attaches to those entities capable of such agency, of doing right or wrong. To defend such a claim one would have to make explicit the necessary qualities an entity must have in order to be capable of both doing wrong and being wronged.

Traditional morality has taken the approach that the highest moral status attaches to human beings. Since such traditional approaches usually sit within a theological framework they have emphasized the role of divine ordination in conferring moral status. Hence, being human is both necessary and sufficient for moral status. When John Harris wrote *The Value of Life* (1985), he did so shortly after the establishment of the Committee of Inquiry into Human Fertilization and Embryology, the so-called 'Warnock Committee'. This government committee was commissioned to inquire into the ethical implications of *in vitro* fertilization (IVF) and related research. Discussions inevitably focused on the moral status of the human embryo and the Catholic Church voiced the traditional view that the embryo had the same inviolable status as any other human being. However, the issues were also aired in secular terms and Mary Warnock, philosopher and chair of the committee argued that:

> 'Human' is a biological term, and simply distinguishes humans from other animals. And it seems to me of paramount importance that we, being human should recognise that there are ways of treating our fellow humans that are right and other ways that are wrong. This is a moral principle, the very principle, in fact, upon which the demand for rights depends.
>
> (Warnock 1983: 241)

By this, Warnock implies that by being human we necessarily partake of humanity, which constitutes a moral domain. As an acknowledged supporter of in vitro fertilization and embryo research Harris rejects this view (Harris 1983). Harris's contribution to the debate is to deny any necessary connection between being human and having moral status. Claims to the contrary he dismisses as 'species prejudice, arbitrary but understandable' (1983: 224). Harris argues that moral status must be independent of any arbitrary ties to species and, hence, he begins to cleave the notion of the person away from that of the human. What constitutes a person for Harris is developed in two parts; first he cites with approval Locke's definition of person quoted above.

Harris approves of Locke's definition of person, for while most human beings are *persons*, no human is a *person* by virtue of their humanity. Harris also approves of the flexibility of Locke's account. Since Locke's criteria are species non-specific they are compatible with the possibility of non-human persons. The as-yet-to-be proven existence of extraterrestrials, who may, in the event, prove to be both alien creatures and alien *persons*. Closer to home, Locke's criteria entertain the possibility of terrestrial non-human *persons*, in the form of non-human animals. Furthermore, given Locke's emphasis on abstract properties it is possible, in principle, for a *person* to be disembodied and, therefore, possible for complex machines to possess the right properties and, hence, have personhood (Harris 1999: 303).

In addition to Locke's account Harris adds the *valuing* criterion. The valuing criterion consists of the capacity to value one's life, for whatever reason; even if an individual values their life negatively they are deemed to have the relevant capacity. So the pre-eminent moral being is the full-blown *person*, a being that has rationality, self-consciousness and the capacity to value its own life (Harris 1985: 14–18). This contrasts with the traditional moral view, which, as I have argued, is consistent with palliative care philosophy and does not require a human being to have such capacities in order to count morally.

Harris's account has far-reaching implications, with consequences for ethics at all stages of the human life span. Even though the primary interest in this book is the end of life I shall, for reasons that will become clear, discuss these consequences with regard to issues at the beginning of life first.

The arguments presented in *The Value of Life* came at a time of wide debate over the ethics of IVF and embryo research. The *person* argument has very specific implications for IVF, embryo research, and for abortion and neonatal care. Harris writes, that on the basis of his argument:

> ... the prospect of concluding that the embryo shares the rights and protections of normal adult human beings is vanishingly small.
>
> It will also be a consequence of the arguments developed here that since neonates and very young children are not capable of wishing to live, it will be no more wrong to kill them, side effects apart, than to kill other creatures of comparable capacities like dogs and sheep.
>
> (Harris 1983: 226)

Harris concludes that the object of his argument, destructive research on the embryo is, by parity of reasoning morally equivalent to the widely accepted practises of contraception and abortion. In all of these cases, Harris argues, nothing of moral worth is destroyed. Harris believes we ought to make the shift from thinking in terms of the anthropocentric person to the abstracted *person* and, in doing so, see the way to unburdening ourselves of some seemingly profound moral problems, destructive embryo research, abortion and various forms of euthanasia. This is, of course, to unfairly condense into a few sentences arguments that have been made over several decades. My point, however, is that by using the approach to ethics, which I have used Harris's work to illustrate, it is possible to see that such arguments imply that ethics has more precision than I believe ethics is capable of. A consequence of accepting the precision claim is the illusion that difficult moral problems can be definitively resolved.

On the face of it Harris does acknowledge that there are some concerns over the precision of his theory:

> The problem is that we not only want reliable criteria for personhood, but we want detectable evidence of personhood. Here matters are not so simple, and we should err on the side of caution and assume, in the case of the sorts of creatures that we know to be normally capable of developing self consciousness, namely human creatures, that they are persons at some safe time prior to the manifestation of the symptoms of personhood. I do not have a set view as to when an appropriate point would be, but I do not think it plausible to regard the emerging human individual, for example, as possessing the relevant capacities at any time while in utero or during the neonatal period.
>
> (Harris 1999: 304–305)

For an account that errs on the side of caution out of concerns for reliability, then this cautious approach still seems rather precise extracting, as it does, from the corpus of moral concerns a whole swathe of issues that seem intuitively to be archetypes of moral problems. Here, I would level the second charge that the *persons* approach yields moral verdicts too far out of line with everyday morality and, in doing so, offends intuition. Of course, the argument from intuition is not itself straight forward. When faced with a counter-intuitive claim in ethics there are two options, we either question and challenge the intuition, and retain or abandon the intuition, or we reject the claim. I shall submit that, in this instance, we reject the claim.

Valuing and attachment

The common thesis of the *persons* approach to ethics is that only some human beings are members of the class of *persons* and this, in so far as they have a capacity for self-valuing. Hence, a morally significant entity is that which is, minimally, capable of holding a value position with regard to itself. Harris tells us:

> I believe those rather simple, even formal features of what it takes to be a person — that persons are beings capable of valuing their own lives — can tell us a good deal about what it is to treat someone as a person.
>
> (Harris 1985: 16)

The fact that I value my life raises the question of whence comes my capacity to value? Harris gives no account of how such a capacity evolves; instead, he leads us to believe, implausibly in my view, that the self-valuer springs forth spontaneously, once a certain threshold of cognitive and linguistic ability is attained. This simplifies a process that is much more subtle and significant in the evolution of the moral agent.

A feature of human offspring is their prolonged dependency as they develop their intellectual and communicative capacities. That adults are usually enchanted by the helplessness of a baby is no doubt an evolutionary trait necessary for survival. However, the nurturing of a child is also a time of rich reciprocal communication with much being expressed behaviourally and non-verbally. We have certainly not exhausted all there is to know about this aspect of human life. To ignore the context in which individuals evolve and are nurtured into adulthood is to ignore an important aspect of human moral evolution.

When Wittgenstein states: 'the human face is the best picture of the human soul' (1958: II. Iv. 178) I take him not to be making a theological claim but rather that the human face, and for that matter the human body, is capable of showing, through its demeanour and through facial expression, instantly recognised by others, the mutuality that is part of our capacity to recognise who and what we are (Wittgenstein 1958). In claiming that it is only in virtue of being a self-valuer that we are able to recognize the value of others, Harris reverses the direction of the relationship between the other and the self, a point hinted at by Adam Smith:

> Where it possible that a human creature could grow up in some solitary place without any communication with his own species, he could no more think of his character, of the propriety or demit of his sentiments and conduct, of the beauty or deformity of his mind, than of the beauty of his own face ... Bring him into society and he is immediately provided with the mirror which he wanted before.
>
> (Smith 1759: III.i.3)

Smith is quoted by Laurence Thomas, who, in a brief discussion of moral psychology, offers an account of the evolution of the self-valuer in the context of human development (Thomas 2000). Thomas claims quite feasibly, that it is in the context of human parental nurturing that the individual develops a sense of both self-worth and the worth of others. Thomas argues that it is through the long process of infant dependency in which the infant's discomforts and insecurities are soothed by its caring parents does it become gradually aware of its own comfort and security and, hence, of self-value. He continues:

> ... what is involved in bringing it about that a child has a sense of intrinsic self-worth is having the experience of being treated in the appropriate way by those who themselves have worth, and so have regard for themselves. From the moral point of view, the intrinsic self-worth that parental love bestows upon the child is what underwrites the child's sense of how he or she should be treated by others.
>
> (Thomas 2000: 152)

I would add to Thomas's account that the nurturing of the child also occurs within a cultural and social context each of which makes a contribution, both to the capacity for valuing and the values that are upheld. Of course, I do not wish to claim too much on the basis of what can only be discussed briefly here. I merely suggest that the experience of being valued and, hence, a sense of self-value is quite plausibly prior to the linguistic abilities needed to conceptualize this status, the basis from which we will stake our claims and make our moral arguments. By comparison to this richer anthropomorphic account, Harris's and other *person*-based accounts appear quite thin.

I suggest that something like the Thomas account comes nearer to the truth of the matter about the background conditions from which a self-valuer evolves. It also offers a picture that is coherent with a more intuitive conception of human value. Harris's characteristics of the person are abstract; in particular, they are not tied to a body or located within a social context. Indeed, in principle, the *person* is entirely separable from the body. On this view, I am a person and presumably would continue to be the same person if the thinking aspect of me was transferred to a dog, cat or Apple Mac. Now, I do not wish to make too much of a possible dualist reading of Harris, but I merely introduce this notion to emphasize the degree to which Harris underestimates the embodied and situated nature of the person. Harris, like other advocates of the *person* approach, has adopted a broadly liberal account of the self, an account that regards the self as existing in isolation, and prior to how it defines itself and its own values, an issue that I will discuss further in relation to the concept of autonomy in chapter 4.

I suggest, contrary to this position, that the person is necessarily embodied and situated, and that this provides a much more authentic model for the human person and the most appropriate starting point for ethics. Wittgenstein's remark suggests that the body is not merely a contingent carrier of the person, but *shows* the person. To see a smile, a wince, a frown in the face of another is to see their satisfaction or discomfort. The expressive and embodied individual is the starting point for moral significance.

The conceptualization of the person as embodied and situated is a familiar one in phenomenological approaches to ethics. Emmanuel Levinas's ethics reflects a central interest of phenomenology: the particular salience of the experience of another person — the Other (Levinas 1989). For Levinas the most salient aspect of this encounter with the Other is the face, since it is the face of the Other, which intrudes upon one's own being with a moral force. For Levinas, the Other is an intrusion into one's own being, experienced not as a presence or an object of knowledge, but as a moral demand not to harm, a moral obligation. The Levinas face is clearly an abstraction, it is not a particular face, but a challenge, it is the vulnerability of the Other that undermines one's own ambitions and ends because it presents us with the potential of obligation or duty.

> The proximity of the other is the faces meaning, [...] Prior to any particular expression and beneath all particular expressions, there is nakedness and destitution of expression as such, that is to say extreme exposure, defencelessness, vulnerability itself. This extreme exposure — prior to any human aim — is like a shot 'at point blank range'
> (Levinas 1989: 83)

What seems apposite to the present discussion is the idea that recognizing the vulnerability of another is also central to human moral experience.

What I have intended by reflecting upon alternative approaches to understanding the human person is to show not only that Harris's account of the person is too thinly drawn, but also that we should be guarded in our approach both to traditional morality and to the overly criteria-based approach of consequentialism and *persons*-based approaches.

So what is my approach to ethics and how will I be deliberating on the issues contained within this book? I am a moral pragmatist and, as such, stand in line with such thinkers as William James and John Dewey, although there are elements of the pragmatic approach evident in many thinkers from Aristotle, to Mill, and more contemporary philosophers. The appeal of pragmatism is its coherence, but also that it allows for the shades of grey that make room for a range of approaches to the sorts of moral problem under consideration. Pragmatism is also consistent with the presumption of moral fallibility as I believe it is wiser to proceed in ethics on the basis that one may need to revise one's position. Before moving on I shall briefly outline what I see as the pragmatic approach to ethics, and in this I am influenced by an essay by Hugh LaFollette (2000). In outlining this approach, I shall also comment upon its particular relevance to the issues to be discussed in this book.

Moral pragmatism

The point of ethics must be practical, since ethics is the evaluation of what we do and how we ought to act. Ethical theory must therefore be relevant to practice and the basic starting point for pragmatic philosophy is that theory is relevant only in so far as it has practical implications. This, I take it, is a point that needs little elaboration in the case of ethics. However, there is a need to give some account of what is meant by pragmatic theory and what is meant by practice in this context. Ethics is awash with theories and, in this chapter, I have outlined traditional 'deontological' ethics, consequentialist ethics, and alluded also to liberalism and phenomenology. However, pragmatism is not a theory in the way that utilitarianism is a theory, but rather pragmatism is a view about how theory is approached. The practice within which theory engages can be characterized in terms of 'habit'. Let me say something about theory first before elaborating what I mean by habit. LaFollette (2000) puts it this way: traditional forms of ethics tend to be absolutist and we have discussed this in terms of the traditional ethical position with regards to the *absolute* sanctity of life, for example, the view that all innocent life is inviolate irrespective of whether a person is aware that they are alive or, indeed, if aware, whether they value their life. Pragmatism attempts to be objective without being absolutist and, in doing so, recognizes that moral judgements are relative, but without being relativistic. This means that there is scope for acknowledging a range of moral positions without accepting that all moral positions are equally justifiable. To avoid the latter conclusion, pragmatic ethics applies criteria without itself being criterial in the way that most ethical theories are. What does 'criterial' mean? A theory is criterial if it accepts some or all of the following; that the criteria of the theory are:

- logically prior (*a priori*);
- unchanging;
- exhaustive;
- directly applicable (LaFollete 2000: 401).

Earlier in this chapter I briefly described Bentham and Mill's utilitarianism, and this provides a relevant example. Although utilitarianism has an empirical component, the thesis that the good life consists of a life in which utility is maximized, is a thesis thought to be true *a priori*, is claimed to be universally true, exhaustive and directly applicable to specific cases. The same charge can be made against deontologists and also of the implicit theory associated with the *persons* approach to ethics. By contrast, the pragmatic approach uses criteria like tools to point to the morally relevant features of action, something that is linked to the necessity of adopting a reflexive and deliberative approach to the features people ought to take into account when making moral judgements. Not that every morally significant action requires a process of deliberation, much of what we do in our moral behaviour is done without deliberation in the same way that our interaction with the physical world is not based upon a need to conduct a continuous empirical enquiry before we place a tentative foot out of bed, this would be to over-rationalize the everyday. Deliberation is needed when we experience a challenge to our personal or collective 'customs' or when our habits fall short of what a new situation demands.

It is understandable to think of habits as unthinking, blind reflexes, that just happen automatically, but this is wrong. As LaFolette puts it, habits have four important elements, they are influenced by our past social experience, they are not simple behaviours, but orchestrated complexes, habits are typically exhibited across a range of circumstances and, even when they are not exhibited, they remain as latent capacities. There are, of course, many kinds of habit from walking, thinking, being musical, acting kindly. The example I cited from Thomas (2000) provides a more complex exemplar of the heritability of habit. How a child is nurtured will influence the child's habit of valuing themselves. How a child is reared will influence how they rear their own children. This is not to say that this happens in a direct and determinate way, habits are empowering, but they are also restrictive, and there is a fine line between being the blind creature of habit, and stepping back from them, evaluating them and attempting to change them.

As a pragmatist I also believe that morality is a habit; a claim that is not quite as remarkable as it may at first appear. For example, not every moral action we perform is the result of conscious deliberation and application of the right criteria. Some of our responses are automatic, we see a person as distressed and we respond in the way that we are habitually disposed to do. One does not, as a rule, *decide* to be kind or empathic — one simply does it. Of course, one can deliberately set out to influence moral habits and I have described elsewhere a process of 'moral' education, which seeks to influence the moral habits of health professionals (Woods 2005). This process, among other things, involves enabling the individual to map the moral domain, establish the 'givens' of moral action and skill the individual in such a way as to render them habitually sensitive to the interests of others.

In conjunction with a deepening moral awareness, there must also be an evolving disposition to act morally together with a capacity for reflexivity. By reflexivity, I mean the capacity to engage in a process of reflection, making aware to oneself the processes involved in making a judgment, and turning such judgment into action with the purpose of reinforcing or revising those processes. This is a critical capacity and is a capacity that can be expressed not just by an individual, but by a society.

To understand how we gain moral habits requires an account of moral epistemology, the process of practical moral reasoning and the objectivity of judgement in relation to the goals of morality. What are the goals of morality? Well, consistent with the pragmatic account, there is no exhaustive account of such goals or ends, but that does not mean that we have no account at all. As with all habits, we learn from our personal and collective experience. Human experience has furnished us with knowledge enough to begin to shade in, with quite some detail, the range of harms and benefits associated with the advance or thwarting of people's interests. There is a useful, if cautiously drawn, analogy here with knowledge in the context of the natural sciences. The lack of a Grand Unifying Theory or our lack of a complete knowledge of matter does not undermine the ability of the natural sciences to provide 'good enough' explanations of the physical world, nor does it mean that the endeavour to seek such a theory, or pursue such knowledge are not useful and important enterprises. I do not believe that moral philosophy is concerned with uncovering new moral 'facts', but is rather concerned with the deepening and enriching of our moral understanding. To claim that there are such goals and goods as flourishing and equality does not require us to give a substantive account of them in advance, since the process of shading in the detail of such goods, the process of rejecting or accepting different accounts of them is itself a process by which our understanding is deepened and enriched (Taylor 1990). The process of reflective deliberation is one process by which moral habits can be improved. As I have argued, reflective deliberation is a process that can be reiterated and engaged with at many levels from individual introspections to more collective deliberations, a process by which a new nuance or layer of insight can be brought to moral understanding. The questioning and challenge of the established boundaries to certain moral habits has in some cases advanced the 'baseline' to the extent that the new parameter becomes the presumed position from which we start, both in terms of personal behaviour and the values that underpin wider social institutions (Moody-Adams 1999). This is not to say that progress is inevitable, but, as Thomas Nagel comments, progress starts with something's having become established as 'obvious' and our setting out begins from there (Nagel 1986). We can see this manifested in contemporary conceptions of moral concepts, such as 'equal respect'. The 'set' to which this moral category applies has been expanded from a position in which women were unquestionably *excluded* to a position where women are unquestionably *included* or, at least, the presumption is now against those whose behaviour reflects the narrower boundary.

Although the boundaries of equal respect have been extended in one direction to the point where contraction is almost inconceivable, the boundaries are not immutable. The frontiers of contemporary moral debate are characterized by disputes as to whether the boundaries can be redrawn in such a way that constitutes a superior set of discriminations, and there are many such boundaries which are relevant to palliative care and end-of-life decisions. Respect for autonomy and the sanctity of life have both influenced and been used to articulate the habits of caring within palliative care. However, the experience of providing care for terminal illness has revealed tensions between these precepts and internal inconsistencies within each. Hence, one of the key questions arising from reflection upon the nature of care at the end of life is whether caring and killing could ever be reconciled in such a way so as to give an 'improved' understanding of what it is to care?

The process by which we may come to such an understanding is complex, if we should reach a point of accepting a new understanding it would not be through a single ethical argument, or by the passing of a particular law, it would be because we have been, as Charles Taylor puts it: '... convinced that a certain view is superior because we have lived a transition which we understand as error-reducing and hence as epistemic gain' (Taylor 1990: 72).

To be convinced by this, we must look not only to the robustness of our arguments, but also to the way in which this new understanding coheres with the rest of moral knowledge, can be incorporated into our moral practises and accommodated by our social institutions. The judgement that leads us to accept a new understanding of a moral practice does not follow from an abstract moral theory, but from our knowledge of harm and suffering, and how to respond to it; it is the practises that give substance to our moral concepts and not the reverse. So it is by taking a pragmatic approach that I turn to consider some of the conceptual and some of the particular ethical issues associated with palliative care and end-of-life decisions.

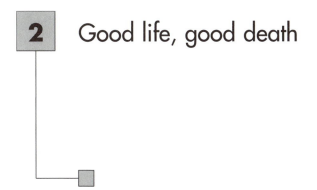

2 Good life, good death

Introduction

Much has been written about the good death. Aries (1976), in a historical study, has suggested that in the West there has been a move from the certainty and solidarity of a shared religious faith to uncertainty, individualism and death denial (Kubler-Ross 1969; Walter 1991; Bauman 1997). It is perhaps unremarkable that the culture of death should have changed given that the contexts and causes of death have altered. Walter (2003) characterizes this as a move from the certainty of a relatively quick death to infectious disease, in the home and under the eye of the priest, to a protracted dying, by chronic disease, within a number of institutions and overseen by a variety of professionals.

Some have seen the development of the hospice movement in terms of an attempt to regain some of the value, and perhaps some of the certainty of the good death. Seale (1989) characterizes one version of the hospice good death ideal as:

> ... getting to know the patients as individuals, treating the family as the unit of care, allowing patients and family to express their needs and preferences, then exercise control over events during their care.
>
> (Seale 1989: 553)

Other commentators have rejected this and similar ideal end-of-life aspirations in favour of alternative models — the least worst death, or the good enough death, the personally ideal death, and the quality of life until death (Battin 1994; McNamara 1998; Randall and Downie 1999). The message is that there is not, and perhaps can never be, a singularly adequate account of the good death in a heterogeneous world (Sandman 2005). Death denial, fragmentation of faiths, fear of death and individualism are leitmotifs of the modern analysis, which relies upon the established dichotomy between the individual and the collective. Exploiting the opposition between the individual and the collective is neat but too simple an analysis. The modern world is sometimes too familiar with the currency of individualism in terms of the person, the consumer and the autonomous agent to also recognize that consumers show trends and agents choose remarkably similar things for themselves when the cards are down. The quest for *personal meaning* has, in the most secular and individualistic societies, become the contemporary euphemism for the spiritual (Walter 1997a), yet in seeking our own personal meaning we forget that if anything has meaning then it is a meaning that can be shared and so, in the end, there is no strictly *personal* meaning. In this book, the tensions between the individual and the collective, between autonomy and responsibility, between the private and the shared will be a continuous theme. However, rather than emphasize the individual and the collective as pulling in opposite directions, I regard them as necessarily entwined, sharing as we do the common ground of culture, society and the fact of human embodiment. To the individual there are some things which seem personal and private to them; their own good death may be one. However, what seems private and individualistic also partakes of common values and exhibits objective qualities, and what can be done to shape the good death is not a private and individual affair either (Field *et al.* 1997).

In this chapter, I take a conceptual approach to exploring the good death with the object of stimulating thoughtful reflection and perhaps even critical rejection of some intuitions of the good death. The conceptual approach employed here uses a method favoured by philosophers, the 'thought experiment'. A thought experiment can be based on realistic, but more often on surrealistic, scenarios in order to explore and clarify common intuitions, testing out the implications of those intuitions often to the point of destruction. Although this chapter can be read as a self-contained discussion of the issues, it also raises questions that will be further explored in subsequent chapters. I offer this reflection on the nature of the good death in the broader context of this book's discussion of palliative care and end-of-life decisions because I believe it has something different to offer in the analysis.

The good death: a thought experiment

Have you ever considered how you would like to die? Some readers may well have not and, for some, even the very question may stir a visceral discomfort; others still will be content with their own acceptance of death. Since we have so far failed to achieve immortality by means either medical or diabolical, then I suggest that this is a good reason to consider the topic at least once.

How we respond to such a question is likely to be influenced, for most of us at least, by the common fears of a negative experience, an undignified end dominated by pain, anxiety and loneliness. However, as an armchair exercise, it is feasible that any one of us might come up with the near ideal scenario. Here is a version of my own.

> I would be very (very) old, reclining in the dappled shade of my apple tree on a perfect English summer's afternoon. I would have just enjoyed a pleasant lunch in the company of my extended family who are continuing to chat around the table. I am in that delicious state of semi-slumber where, although I am aware of the sounds of the outside world, the voices of my family, the happy play of the grandchildren, the drone of an even more distant passing car, all of which come to me as from a great distance. I would be lying with perhaps no more dis-comfort than a stiff neck or dry mouth, but not enough discomfort to make me want to move or seek a drink for fear of losing that delicious moment of somnolence — at which point I slip into unconsciousness and death.

This, of course, is a fantasy, one in which indignity and discomfort are conveniently ignored. It is also a fantasy unlikely to be realized since most people die in hospital or a nursing home in circumstances beyond their control and not in the midst of an extended family (Thorpe 1993). There is the ideal and then there is the reality.

I begin with this question and my own hypothetical answer to it because I wish to explore the nature of the good death and consider the degree to which the good death can be achieved. These reflections are intended as a conscious revival of a long-abandoned but, in my opinion, under-valued tradition of *ars moriendi* — the art of dying well. In this chapter I contrast some contemporary and secular versions to the traditional Christian version by exploring the characteristics and qualities of the good death.

The ideal death scenario sketched above is but one version of a type, the slipping-peacefully-away at the end of a long and successful life. This is an idealized human story, but one that many will identify with. There are, of course, many different versions of this type and numerous variations on this theme of the good death (Sandman 2005). For many of us, the chances of achieving our own version of a good death will not be realized because our options will be foreclosed by circumstances out of our control. However, given that we, through our own efforts or through the offices of those who manage our deaths, can influence the nature and timing of our death, then we must inevitably turn to the questions of what we ought to be permitted to do or command others to do to achieve this? So the slipping-peacefully-away kind of death will be, but one, perhaps one of the most important types, of the models to be explored.

Even the most rudimentary of reflections on the nature of the good death will quickly make clear that there are certain salient parameters and qualities that matter. Pain, suffering, mental awareness, timing, context and life success are just some of these. I will now turn to identifying and exploring some of these *parameters* of the good death.

Parameters of the good death

The philosopher Wittgenstein once remarked cryptically that 'death is not an event in life' (1958: 193). A practical interpretation of this remark suggests that death is not an experience, unlike other events we experience, because death is not *lived* through. In other words, for something to be experienced as an event in one's life there must be continuity of experience — a before and after experience. This observation is significant, since it establishes one of the important parameters when reflecting upon the nature of the good death, that for the dying person death is not an experience that is lived through, but the dying is. Therefore, experientially speaking, what matters are the events leading up to death and not what happens after death, although if one has a religious faith or is genuinely agnostic then there may, indeed, be anxieties about what happens after death that have an impact on the quality of life before death. For the Christian these sorts of concerns are what influenced the original *ars moriendi*. Clearly, one's preferences for what happens to one's body after death may also be a significant aspect of any of our concerns for the good death. My point here is that, *post-mortem,* this cannot matter experientially. So now I turn to consider other candidates for the good death with a particular focus upon the experiential aspects.

Sudden death

One often hears the remark, either as an observation or an aspiration that to go suddenly, without knowing a thing about it would be a good way to go (Williams 1990; Walter 2003). This hypothesis can, to an extent, be empirically tested by comparing it with the closest experience to sudden death that one can actually experience; that of suddenly fainting. One moment you are standing upright, the next thing you are aware of it is several moments later when coming to, perhaps with a distressed person shaking you into consciousness. Clearly, this is not death; one survives a faint, but it is plausible to presume that all the events leading up to the faint would have been identical had this been a case, not of fainting, but rather of sudden death, except that the temporary interruption of consciousness would have been permanent. Reflecting on this sort of experience suggests that sudden death, with no insight into what is about to occur is, from the perspective of the person experiencing it, a good way to die. There is no frightening anticipation, no suffering and no slow decline; perhaps just a fleeting warning and then nothing.

It is reasonable to conclude, therefore, that an important parameter of a good death is the quality of the dying person's experiences prior to death. So we have one hypothetical ideal, that of the sudden unanticipated death. Of course, this is but one parameter and that has been rather thinly described, since a moment's reflection on this solipsistic version of the good death, quickly gives rise to a different consideration that is also undermining of the ideal. This other consideration is the quality of the experiences of those who survive the death or, more to the point, the experiences of those who care about the deceased.

Death viewed from a third person perspective is an event that *is* lived through by those who witness it. One's sudden and unexpected death would be a very disturbing experience for those close to you. So care must be taken not to over-generalize here. Sudden death that is unexpected may be a *comparatively* better ending for the one who dies, relative to a lingering and painful death, but may be much worse for the survivors. So the quality of one person's death is also reflected in the experiences of others. How others experience a death is quite reasonably another of the salient parameters to add to the developing model of the good death. This is an aspect of dying with which the palliative care community has acknowledged and responded to, forming the basis, as it does, of the palliative care approach to family care, which extends into the period of bereavement after death (Ellershaw and Ward 2003).

Perhaps a sudden death, where death *is* expected, may reasonably be presumed to be a better death than a sudden unexpected death, or an anticipated death that is lingering and also painful. What I mean here is, for example, a person who is terminally ill and is expected to die after several months of slow decline, but due to a sudden and unforeseen event they die suddenly after only a few weeks. For the person who dies it seems better, objectively speaking, because in their lifetime they will have experienced less pain and distress, significant tokens of 'bad' experiences. Nevertheless, a sudden death of this kind may be bad in other ways, depriving the deceased, as well as those left alive of an opportunity to complete the necessarily 'unfinished business' of their life, to round things off and say their goodbyes. The advocates of palliative care also comment that this is a time that offers opportunities for 'continued growth' implying that any foreshortened life is potentially a missed opportunity.

While it makes sense to talk of the quality of dying and death as necessary to a conception of the good death, this is only part of the picture. I have talked so far only of discrete experiences and events, but the meaning and value of these have a context. So judgements of 'good,' 'bad,' 'better,' or 'worse' deaths are not absolutes, but relative to time, place, persons, etc. and the panoply of other human concerns that influence the evaluation of life and death. Dying and death viewed as discrete events at the end-of-life divorces these events from the whole of the person's life, which is their proper context. There is, therefore, an overarching evaluation of death and dying in the broader context of the life of which death marks the end.

There are numerous examples that illustrate the complexity and contrasts that exist in the different evaluations to be made of different kinds of death. Take dying young, for example, one may think that a life taken so prematurely is always a tragedy, but there are differences to be drawn. Contrast the 'James Dean' ending to that of a fragile adolescent, who after her first rejection in love gestures at suicide by taking paracetamol and unintentionally succeeds. The James Dean version of dying young, for all its tragedy has a certain coherence with the image of the young rebel that is absent from the unintended gesture suicide within an immature life. There is a sense in which both kinds of death illustrated here are merely clichés. The suggested evaluation of these deaths is perhaps just one of the many representations of death imposed by cultural stereotypes. However, the intuition these examples are intended to provoke here is a relatively simple one. Of all the possible kinds of death that might be ours there is a sense in which a death that is consistent, and coherent with the kind of life we sought to live is a better death for this consistency. The death of Cicely Saunders, who died in the hospice she helped to found, in receipt of the care she helped to pioneer, might be illustrative of the thought that the evaluation of a death is framed by the life in which it has a context. Or, to use a different example, the death of Rob Hall, a high altitude mountain guide, who died on his return from the summit of Everest when he was caught in a now famously violent storm in which many climbers died. Hall died because he tried to save a client struggling in the storm and, although his death was a tragedy, dying in the place and the way he did, one can speculate, had a coherence with the rest of his life, which had he been killed crossing the road, would not. So the idea of the consistency of a death with the rest of a life suggests that a further parameter of the good death, at least at a simple intuitive level, is that of coherence. I use this guarded form of expression because I realize that the concept of coherence is complex as Sandman (2005) demonstrates in his interesting treatment of the concept.

If we, for example, ask who judges the coherence of a death, then this is one way in which this complexity is revealed. How I might judge my death in anticipation may be very different from how my loved ones judge it. Widening the perspective still further to the public gaze then the death of a 'villain', who lived by the sword and died by the sword, may be judged coherent from the perspective of natural justice; 'he got what he deserved', but not necessarily from his own perspective. These complexities aside, I suggest that there is a sense in which coherence matters and when this cannot be achieved then second best is the avoidance of gross inconsistency.

The idea that coherence is a quality of the good death has been echoed by other writers. For some it is seen as a feature that emphasizes individual differences, Saunders writes: '... it soon became clear that each death was as individual as the life that preceded it and the whole experience of that life was reflected in a patient's dying'. (Saunders 1996: 1600). For others, it is a positive aspiration, an expression of individuality and autonomy, indeed, a moral right that enables a person to shape the end of their life in a manner consistent with the rest of their life (McNamara 1998). For Dworkin (1993) the idea of coherence is closely tied to personal autonomy and the integrity that autonomy brings to a life, writing in support of the role of advance directives in determining the nature of one's dying he comments:

> Making someone die in a way that others approve, but he believes a horrifying contradiction of his life, is a devastating, odious form of tyranny.
>
> (Dworkin 1993: 217)

Although I have suggested a number of ways in which we can understand coherence, which conception we choose will have implications for how we value coherence as an attribute of a life. Is coherence valuable because of the coherence we impose upon our own lives or because of some objective view of the coherence of our life we ourselves maybe did not see? The quote from Ronald Dworkin above suggests that we make our own lives coherent from the autonomous control we have over our lives, and in Dworkin's view this gives the best reason to respect individual autonomy. However, the version of autonomy this implies, with its inherent tendency to downgrade all other interests in favour of autonomy is itself also contested (Dresser 1995). Coherence of this kind is perhaps valued precisely because, for a person like Dworkin, autonomy is so highly prized, but as Sandman (2005) points out this may become less emphatically the case when an individual finds themselves in new circumstances and facing a particularly challenging situation as so frequently happens when a person finds themselves in terminal decline. Sandman makes two further points, the first is that a death may be judged 'good' even at the price of a previously consistent and strongly held value; so coherence is not strictly necessary for a good death. Sandman's second point is that there can be no obligation imposed on carers to provide a death that is coherent for the patient where this requires injustice to other patients in terms of use of resources or else clashes with the other normative values of health care practice. So in seeking to describe the 'good' making features of the good death one must be cautious to distinguish the intuitively plausible parameters from a normative set of requirements, which may impose a duty on society, the family or professional carers.

In summary, when thinking abstractly of the nature of the good death there are a number of intuitively plausible parameters:

- the quality of the experiences of the dying person;
- the quality of the experiences of third parties;
- the timing of the death;
- the coherence of the death with the rest of the person's life.

In these few simple examples we have begun to characterize, but clearly not exhaust, an *axiology* of dying.

Axiology and the good death

Axiology is the philosophical approach to theorizing about the good life. Axiology is primarily the study of the formal elements of the good life and is not to be confused with contemporary notions of quality of life, which is generally an empirical discipline (Parfit 1991; Bowling 1995). This said, many quality of life measures are, to varying degrees, premised upon philosophical theories. Axiology is neither concerned with *moral* goodness, although inevitably there is a sense in which the pursuit of the good life must be justified in moral terms.

If axiology is the theory of the good life is it plausible to talk of the good death in the context of axiology? I shall argue that it is since the goodness of a life must take into account the whole of a life, and therefore the end is as significant as the beginning or any other aspect that shapes a life. Death and, indeed, dying are necessary components of an account of the good life, since the latter marks the final experiences of life, and the former the end of the life. The character of one's death and dying can therefore be seen to be significant, *when* one dies and *how* one dies may influence the judgement of the overall goodness of one's life and not just the final moments.

The parallel between the good life and the good death again raises a key question, the possibility of shaping the goodness of a life? It will be appreciated that, in life, we are born into a set of circumstances, material wealth and social conditions, which set limits on our opportunities. We are also exposed to the vicissitudes of fate, what some have called 'moral luck'. In other words, things happen to us that may be good or bad for us, and these factors are largely out of our control. However, some of these are things we can control and, endeavouring to live a better life, many people attempt to exert control over factors that in the past were accepted fatalistically. What we accept as given and what we regard as open to our influence is not fixed, and this naturally poses the question of what importance we attach to what is given, and what it is permissible to manage and influence?

The four parameters of the good death described so far, taken in the abstract, are the sort of *formal* characteristic with which axiology is concerned. There are, of course, limits to what can be said on the basis of formal characteristics, it is not plausible to offer a substantive account of the good life or death; nevertheless the qualities of experience, timing and coherence have a useful function, they are 'good making' factors that form part of a framework. In chapters 4 and 5, I will explore axiology in more detail when discussing the concept of autonomy and its relevance to palliative care. For now, I shall turn to the task of exploring the good death through an axiological framework.

Individual deaths may be timely or untimely, experientially good or bad, and because different people value different things, good and bad in many different ways. However, although the specifics will vary according to individual lights the theoretical 'shape' of a good life/death can be characterized within an abstract framework, and in using the concept of axiology I shall begin to explore some plausible 'shapes'.

There are two broad theoretical approaches to axiology: one that gives priority to essentially subjective accounts of the good life and the other, which gives a broadly objective account of the good life. Both approaches have a strong intuitive appeal and sit well with the parameters already discussed (Griffin 1986; Brock 1993; Nussbaum and Sen 1993; Sandman 2005)

According to Brock (1993) subjective theories are primarily concerned with either the quality of one's experiences or with one's preferences, and their satisfaction. Theories of the good life that focus on the quality of experiences, are concerned with experiences in terms of the way they feel for the person having them, in other words, a better life is a life in which there are more good experiences than bad experiences. This version of an axiology is itself consistent with the experiential aspects of dying we have considered so far.

Hedonism is the philosophical theory that gives priority to experiential aspects when evaluating a life. Hedonism, as described within classical utilitarianism, is the theory that a good life is a life lived in the pursuit of pleasure, broadly construed and the avoidance of pain. In terms of making a broad hedonistic evaluation of the 'goodness' of a life, this can be done in either a positive or negative way, and again this seems to cohere with some basic intuitions. If construed negatively, the goodness of a life is judged in terms of the avoidance of bad experiences and there follows some very practical implications for end-of-life care. In the context of palliative care Randall and Downie (1999) describe an important objective of palliative care as the intention: 'to manoeuvre the illness along the least unpleasant course and about enabling the patient to die of their illness in the least unpleasant way' (1999: 174). So the negative hedonistic model offers an account of the good death, which is consistent with at least one approach to palliative care.

A challenge for hedonism, as for any adequate theory of the good life, is the task of explaining the place of experiences such as pleasure and pain in a way that is not overly simplistic, that gives weight to different kinds of experience not only in terms of their quality, but also in terms of what they mean for the person having them. A theory that gives weight to the seeking and avoidance of certain experiences needs to say something about how we attach meaning to such experiences within the context of a whole life, otherwise hedonism seems unconvincing as a complete account of the good life.

Pain, for example, seemingly the obvious token of a bad experience, is in reality much more ambiguous. Even severe pain, may be endured for the sake of some important and realizable good, quite meaningfully captured in the old adage about the benefits of physical training, 'no pain, no gain'. Researchers have frequently described how, in different contexts, the meaning of pain endows it with a relative value, for example, people seem to be able to endure in the context of a religious rite what would otherwise be a painful mutilation (Melzack and Wall 1988). If one compares, for example, the pain associated with childbirth with the pain associated with torture and the very different impact these experiences have on the life of the individual, then the range and complexity of pain can be appreciated, if only theoretically, by most of us.

Many people might be sympathetic to the idea that a life can be described as good or bad in character relative to the degree of pain a person suffers, or the other bad experiences an individual has. However, even this seemingly obvious claim requires cautious qualification. For example, even if we limit the class of 'bad' experiences to painful physical sensations then it is not at all obvious that pain or suffering can be summed so as to make comparisons of better or worse meaningful. If I have experienced 10 severe pains for 30 years, is it objectively the case that my life is worse than that of my brother who experienced merely mild discomfort only once per week? As I have suggested, it is impossible to separate the *experience* from the life and meaning that gives it context. What if my pain were linked to my aspiration to excel on the parallel bars, whereas my brother felt profoundly depressed because his discomfort interfered with his watching of daytime TV? The problems of making inter-life comparisons are profound ones; however, if everyone restricts judgement to one's own life then the claim that life goes better, relatively speaking, if there are fewer bad experiences like pain, seems reasonable, but on closer scrutiny it is far more complex. If, for example, I could stand outside of my life in a position from where it was possible to 'look down' so to speak, from an objective position, then would I be able to sum the quality of experiences for myself over a lifetime? This abstract approach only serves to reveal that the complexity, pains and pleasures are meaningless without the context of the life in which they occur.

Hedonist theory becomes more challenging when one attempts to reconcile the relationship between good and bad experiences. The point hinges on whether good and bad experiences are relative to one another or whether good and bad experiences belong to a distinct class? To pull experiences apart in this way seems artificial, for example, the reduction of pain might also be judged to be an enhancement. One might equally argue that hedonism ought to give positive weight to 'good' experiences. Positive hedonism might be premised upon the idea that a life goes best if one aims to positively enhance that life with good experiences in addition to minimizing bad ones. Applying this account to the context of the good death then, the negative version of hedonism might suggest that a good death can itself be negatively characterized in terms of the absence of adverse symptoms, pain, cramps, nausea or depression, anxiety and so on. Positive hedonism suggests that, in order to achieve a good death, it is legitimate, required even, to deliberately enhance the experiences of the dying person in a positive way. So that the good death is characterized not merely as an absence of symptoms, but in terms of somehow enhanced, or 'improved' physical and mental states. Christian axiology in the form of *ars moriendi* emphasized the importance of certain mental states, awareness and preparedness, a contrite mind and one ready to fend off temptation. These are mental states valued because of their place within a particular system of belief. However, alertness, clarity of mind, reconciliation and acceptance are mental qualities commonly described as elements within contemporary accounts of good dying, without implying necessarily, any religious values or beliefs, yet in their own way equally value laden (Kubler-Ross 1969; McNamara *et al.* 1994). Cicely Saunders (1969), for example, when advocating the judicious use of opiates, sedatives and even alcohol in terminal care, comments upon the importance of avoiding their 'stuporose' effects. This implies that there is a distinction to be drawn between different mental states, some which may be regarded as good, in and of themselves, some which may be regarded as instrumental to other valuable ends and others that are neither good nor desirable yet may be 'tolerated' as necessary side-effects; and still some which are seen as unequivocally bad. This approach begins to suggest a means to discriminate between the proper goals of treatment and care and those which can be seen as falling outside of the range.

When thinking about the goal of achieving a good death, and the experiential components specifically, there is also a possible moral asymmetry to be drawn between 'good' and 'bad' experiences. This is clearer if 'good' and 'bad' experiences are construed in terms of pleasure and pain. Pain has the potential to create a moral claim that pleasure does not. In health care ethics, there is often talk of a duty not to inflict pain or an obligation to relieve pain if we can. This has become enshrined in the Hippocratic medical ethical duty of 'do no harm'. The same emphasis is not given to a possible parallel duty to give pleasure or enhance the quality of a person's experiences. The nearest equivalent is perhaps the duty of beneficence; to do some positive good, but this is usually in the context of curing or palliating harm, and not of enhancement. In the medical context enhancement, at least above the norm, is regarded as supererogatory, and in many medical fields the blurring of the boundary between treatment and enhancement is regarded as a wrong. To be sure the picture is more complex than the sketch I offer here. The duty to 'do good' in a medical sense might realistically be construed in terms of improving quality of life, which is measured not only in an objective functional sense, but also includes subjective states expressed in terms of 'well-being' (Boddington and Podpadec 1992). In palliative care the goal of achieving a good death has, as Randall and Downie (2006) observe, itself been subsumed in a broader attention to quality of life (World Health Organization (WHO) 2002). An analysis of the goals and purposes of medicine in terms of the duty to do good may be characterized in different ways. Doing good may be construed negatively, to palliate or slow the process of deterioration, or it may be regarded positively as curing or improving function in which improvements in well-being are regarded as a beneficial side-effect. Improvements in welfare aimed at, but as a secondary goal, are impossible to separate within the cause and effect of treatment, a recognition of the holistic nature of health and well-being. Finally, merely aiming to make a person 'feel' better independently of a cure or improved functionality would be regarded as unethical where improved function or cure were themselves realistic goals.

There is a long history in western culture that regards the pursuit of pleasure as morally suspect. In the context of enhancing pleasurable experiences specifically in the medical context then this notion might well be regarded as dubious, non-medical and abusive even, blurring the distinction between substance use and abuse, for example. However, the idea of positively enhancing experiences, while seemingly suspect might, in fact, have a respectable place within the goals of palliative care.

I therefore raise the question, in the context of this axiological enquiry, could hedonistic enhancement be regarded as instrumental to a good death? Should palliative care embrace a form of positive hedonism and aim to enhance the dying person's experiences? If so what boundaries might be imposed upon both the degree and the means of such enhancement?

This is difficult ground, but consider first the plausibility of the claim that deliberately aiming to induce a positive change in the experiences of the dying person might be a legitimate goal of palliative care. I shall begin by suggesting a number of ways in which this 'obvious outrage' might not seem so scandalous. First, there is no question that one of the first concerns for the early palliative care movement was the adequate treatment for symptoms and the adequate treatment of pain being the highest priority. Pain relief in terminal care came in the form of morphine or an elixir whose basic ingredients might include morphine, cocaine, alcohol and chloroform, the so-called 'Brompton's cocktail', all of which are drugs used recreationally for their 'pleasant' effect, although it would be distorting the truth to suggest that the primary use of such substances was this effect. The use of narcotics might be construed entirely within the negative hedonistic model outlined above, but other goals may not. The palliative care objective to improve quality of life cannot be easily classified as a negative 'good,' although aiming to enhance the quality of life of a terminally ill person may be justified in terms of attempting to restore the patient to somewhere near the norm, rather than by aiming to enhance them beyond it. Contemporary palliative care services have extended to include not only terminal care, but respite care, rehabilitation and day hospice care, with an emphasis on providing a range of complementary therapies, the purposes of which cannot be construed solely in terms of treatment or even of palliation. However, therapies as disparate as massage, aromatherapy and neuro-linguistic programming are aimed at enhancing either through a pleasant physical sensation or through psychological effects, the quality of the experiences as well as the quality of life of the recipient.

Many medications used in the treatment of pain, such as opiates and steroids, have effects that alter the conscious state of the person, changing their perception of the pain by dulling or 'distancing' it, but also by inducing and enhancing other sensations, such as mild euphoria or a feeling of well-being. There has even been speculation and some early research about the possible clinical application of LSD or similar 'psychedelic' drugs in terminal care with a view to enabling the patient to come to a peaceful acceptance of their death (Kurland 1985). Cicely Saunders was herself interested in the possible applications for LSD in terminal care and, in a letter to the editor of *Harper's* Magazine, she writes requesting the contact details of a researcher who had written of his work for the magazine:

> I would like to get in touch with him. What is of particular interest to me is the fact that my patients say something of the same kind of thing about their dying as does the patient he quoted and the vast majority of the hundreds whom I have looked after over the past years have reached their death in a spirit of quiet serenity and acceptance. This is not with the use of LSD but with other drugs which are at present available to any physician and opportunities to give time and an attempt to understand what it feels like to be so ill.
>
> (Clark 2002a: 94)

Alcohol and anxiolytics, in addition to steroids and narcotics, are all staples of the palliative formulary and their use is tolerant of the sometimes beneficial side-effects that are not directly aimed at. Talk of 'tolerated but not directly aimed at' is to offer a secondary or 'double-effect' account of the goal of medicine, which is capable of distinguishing the proper goal of palliative care from the questionable deliberate aim to influence the quality of a person's experiences. The fact that we may intuitively reject such an idea as repugnant helps to throw into relief some of the norms surrounding contemporary ideas of good dying and the good death, and the role of palliative care in this.

However, it might also be argued that deliberately aiming to induce or enhance pleasant experiences is entirely consistent with the goals of palliative care so long as this is within a certain boundary. How might such a boundary be characterized? One of the distinctions that may be useful in circumscribing such a boundary is that between use and misuse; and there are a number of ready-to-hand illustrations.

Consider the following illustration; the mood altering affects of alcoholic drinks, for example, are enjoyed by many people. Those who use alcohol will recognize the benefits of alcohol as an aperitif or as a means of assisting the feeling of bonhomie among dinner guests. Notwithstanding the benefits, most people would not wish to live out their lives in an alcoholic haze; indeed, part of the reason why people enjoy alcohol is because its effect is transient and temporary. We recognize and usually appreciate the difference between being 'under the influence' and not. The ability to make such discriminations is part of the capacity to make a good judgement and is necessary in distinguishing use from misuse. The capacity for this kind of judgement also draws on other valuing concepts such as proportionality and appropriateness, and although these concepts are highly relativistic they are less so when considered in relation to a particular goal. So the use of alcohol to achieve the goal of a successful dinner party will undermine that goal if its use is inappropriate or disproportionate.

From this commonplace example we can derive an approach that is applicable to the consideration of the goals of palliative care, and the appropriate use and misuse of different kinds of treatment in palliative care. Deliberately aiming to alter mental states might therefore be judged appropriate where the patient wants this, the effect is temporary and transient and does not become a dominant end in itself. The concepts of appropriateness and proportionality will be revisited later in this book, for now, I wish to consider a related version of subjective theories of axiology, and connect this to the good death and the boundaries of palliative care. Earlier in this chapter, I commented that the second of the two subjective theories of the good life was that of preference satisfaction. On this view, a good life is good in so far as each individual has their preferences satisfied, and is bad in so far as the satisfaction of preferences is frustrated. Taken at face value, this theory also gives weight to the value of individual autonomy since this allows each person to define their own set of preferences and pursue them. Superficially, at least, this is a theory that seems compatible with many of the practises of palliative care, which attempts to respect the patient and allow them, at least a degree, of choice to determine how they would prefer to live their life to its end.

The philosopher Robert Nozick (1984) challenged the preference satisfaction theory of the good life with his now infamous 'pleasure machine' thought experiment. While there is some disagreement as to whether the argument against preference satisfaction was entirely successful, it does provoke a number of thoughts that are relevant to this discussion. A contemporary version of this experiment might be as follows:

> Imagine that a virtual reality machine has been perfected so that anyone connected to the machine would be unable to distinguish virtual experience from real experience. Imagine further that one could program the machine so that the user might experience any kind of life they desired. Perhaps the life of a brilliant and successful sport star, lionised by an adoring public and with all the plaudits and material wealth that goes with such a life.

If you can suspend disbelief enough to play the game this thought experiment requires, then it is possible to imagine all sorts of applications of this machine. Imagine a terminally ill patient, struggling to come to terms with their imminent death, and doing so without support of friends and family. If the patient were to use the machine, then they might live out their days peacefully accepting death, lovingly supported by friends and family, or by enjoying some other fantasy good life until their death. Now putting yourself in the place of the patient ask yourself why would you *not* plug into the machine?

Perhaps the most obvious reason for not using the machine is that every satisfaction the machine gave would be false. The feelings of pride and joy as the successful sports hero, the feeling of love and support from friends and family for the patient, would not be authentic, even though the experience was completely convincing in how it 'felt', these feelings would be unconnected to reality and therefore false. Although this science-fiction fantasy may seem quite trivial, it does reveal something profound about how we conceive the goodness of a life. Truth, reality and authenticity matter because we want our projects to be successful and not merely for us to be tricked into believing they have been; we want our friendships to be genuine and not merely seem so; and we expect that the decisions we make for ourselves cause things to happen in the real world. This is what I refer to as the 'reality constraint' upon our desire satisfaction.

The relevance to palliative care might seem quite obvious, dealing truthfully and honestly with patients, allowing people to make decisions that have a genuine effect, not employing treatments and therapies that unnecessarily detract from a person's connection with reality and so on. While the implications seem obvious at one level there is another tier of complexity to consider. The way this thought experiment has been set up asks us to consider its implications from the personal, the first person, perspective. How would I feel 'from the inside' if I discovered that my own experiences, relationships and so on were not genuine? From the first person perspective, it is relatively easy to appreciate the obvious objective value of truth and reality in relation to the actual fulfilment of one's preferences, but things are quite different if one is asked to consider the situation of another person. Posing the question from the third person perspective reveals that, while it may be obvious for me that my life goes best if important components of it are authentic and real, does it also follow that this is something that ought to be imposed on others? Put this way, the problem is not that the value of truth and authenticity are diminished, but rather that there is a challenge concerning how we relate to others with respect to these values. It should be obvious that these axiological values pose an ethical problem, particularly in the palliative care context, where a commitment to open communication and acceptance of death are acknowledged goals.

Truth, authenticity and reality can be described as objective characteristics of a good life and, having introduced these, it is appropriate to say something briefly about objective axiological theory.

Good life, good death, good endings

To some, the idea of an objectively good death (just as the idea of an objectively good life) would seem nonsense — and there has been a long tradition of debate on this issue. Much, of course, hinges upon what is meant by 'objective'. I spoke earlier of the possibility of a new *ars moriendi* and described this as a secular, rather than Christian development. The Christian tradition does purport to give an objective account of the good death since it stipulates the terms in which the good Christian soul ought to pass over. So the Christian 'good death' gives an account of both the objective good-making qualities, clarity of mind, clear conscience, and preparedness and the moral imperative, this is what the good Christian ought to do.

The question now is whether a contemporary and secular *ars moriendi* can embrace both the objective qualities and an equivalent moral imperative. While I have begun to outline a number of candidate good-making qualities for the good death, I have not addressed the question of whether there can be anything like a moral imperative to conform to a particular way of dying. Although this is a question that will be returned to throughout the book I will say something briefly now.

The Christian approach, which I have used as an example of a traditional *ars moriendi*, does offer a substantive account of what being a good Christian entails. Being a good Christian was not, of course, only confined to the dying Christian, but applied throughout a life. However, thinking about the good death as a secular *ars moriendi*, this does not draw upon a single corpus of tradition and theology, and therefore cannot offer a substantive positive account of how one ought to live and die. This disquiet has been widely reflected in the critical treatment given to the good death ideals, which have become common currency within the palliative care literature (Hart *et al.* 1998; McNamara 1998; Clark and Seymour 1999). It has been noted that descriptions of the good death were in danger of becoming moral prescriptions and, hence, advancing an ideal that was setting most people up to fail by falling short of the good death ideal. So what are the implications for a contemporary *ars moriendi*? As an alternative to the substantive ideal, there has been a trend towards pragmatic and 'negative' formulations with the 'least worst' death the new substantive goal. Is there a parallel moral imperative? The growth in the importance of individual autonomy has meant that the advocates of autonomy have called for greater freedom for individuals to shape their dying. However, the palliative care community has conceded respect to autonomy only in so far as informed compliance with medical norms or informed refusal of medical interventions can achieve this.

These are important issues that will be addressed by the rest of this book and so now I shall return to axiology and characterizing the parameters of the good death.

Axiological trajectories

There has been a trend in the palliative care literature to employ so-called 'illness trajectories' as conceptual aids to planning future care needs, as well as helping to address with patients and families that most difficult of questions: 'what will happen next?' (Lynn and Adamson 2003, Murray *et al.* 2005). I now wish to employ a similar device, using the trajectory format, to map out some of the intuitions we have begun to explore about the nature of the good life. First, a precautionary note about the limitations of this approach, the trajectories I shall discuss are purely heuristic devices, they are not, as in the case of illness trajectories, based upon any form of empirical evidence. I shall be using the device conceptually, to test out certain intuitions as a continuation of the thought experiment approach employed so far in this chapter. In our earlier discussion, we conclude that there were a number of parameters of the good death:

- the quality of the experiences of the dying person;
- the quality of the experiences of third parties;
- the timing of the death;
- the coherence of the death with the rest of the person's life.

I now want to draw attention to the Figures 2.1 and 2.2.

There are, of course, severe limitations as to what can be represented by a simple two-dimensional diagram. However, the area under the curve (AUC)

Figure 2.1 Axiological templace

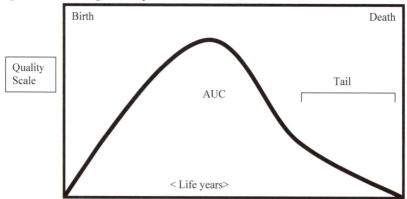

Figure 2.2 Alternative endings

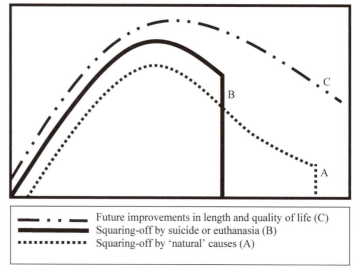

(Figures reprinted with permission from Woods and Elstein (2002))

is, nevertheless, a plausible representation offering a *very* rough template of an idealized *good* life. Let me say in what way the AUC can be seen as representing *a* 'shape' of a good life and suggest how such intuitions pre- dictably differ according to the various points on the life trajectory. For example, consider the area identified as the 'tail' in Figure 2.1. There is a common intuition that the further a life proceeds into the tail, the greater the ambivalence about the meaning and value of the life lived at this time compared with some central point on the trajectory. If the tail equates to a prolonged dwindling (Lynn and Adamson 2003), then this time may be regarded as bad, diminishing the goodness of a life. This observation seems to cohere with other intuitions, such as the intuition implicit within the time trade-off principle, that people would, rather have a shorter life of better quality than a longer life of poor quality (Buxton and Ashby 1988).

I have already attempted to characterize some possible intuitions with regard to life at the tip of the tail. For example, the idea of sudden death is represented in Figure 2.2 by line A, showing a foreshortening of the tail by 'squaring-off' the curve. Out of all the possible endings then, other things being equal, a short period of rapid decline may be preferable to prolonged dwindling. We have already discussed that a sudden death that is unexpected may be a *comparatively* better ending for the one who dies, than a lingering and painful death, but may be much worse for the survivors.

The idea of a *natural* 'squaring-off' also seems consistent with the intuition that supports the time trade-off principle. Of course, the problem with taking this abstract and objective approach is that it removes us as individuals from the reality of the life that is ours. Do we really know how we would feel if we found ourselves having a prolonged slow decline? It has been commented many times that healthy people and health workers particularly underestimate the value of life lived with a chronic disease. A further criticism could be made that to consider possible alternative endings in the abstract is to do so without the knowledge of the kind of death that will be ours. Some advocates of palliative care maintain that the kind of death that one has is and ought to remain a matter of moral luck, that is; whatever happens to befall us. Drawing upon points considered earlier in this chapter, this approach might be seen as consistent with the proper role of palliative care, which should aim to ameliorate, but not to fundamentally change the nature of the 'natural death' that will be ours.

Figure 2.2, by contrast, also represents three alternative endings, which, considered in the abstract explore a number of logical alternatives. The idea that a natural squaring-off, as represented by line 'A', is preferable to a prolonged dwindling, raises the question of whether this is a feature that ought to be engineered by non-natural means? This takes us from a consideration of the range of deaths determined by nature to the possibility of squaring-off by deliberate action; by suicide or assisted death. In the abstract, the possibility of having control over certain 'good-making' features is consistent with the idea that certain parameters such as the timing and the opportunity to plan and finish final tasks are part of a common conception of the good death. I have been careful to premise my comments with 'in the abstract' since for the purposes of the axiological approach taken in this chapter I have suspended the moral dimension. However, the ethical implications of turning the abstract into reality are clear and many people take the view that this is an area of human intervention that should not be endorsed because of the wrongness of killing; an issue I shall take up in chapter 7.

The alternative possibility to squaring-off by killing is that of deep and permanent sedation during the dying phase. If this were possible it would in effect mean achieving a death 'analogue' in which a person is effectively experientially 'dead' before they have reached the tip of the tail. I have already indicated a possible objection to this intervention in the earlier discussion of truth and reality. For some, rendering a person permanently unconscious, in addition to the ethical concerns, may be seen as inconsistent with the 'reality constraint'; that a good death ought to keep a person, as far as possible, in touch with reality.

The final trajectory posited as logically possible is the 'flattened' curve, indicating the possibility of life extension. Of course, if the shape of the trajectory represented in Figure 2.1 were to represent actual life expectancy, then plotting this over recent decades would reveal the transformation the West has undergone over a relatively short period of time.

We are all, at least in the developed world, the beneficiaries of a life extension programme, since most of us now enjoy longer lives of better quality than our recent ancestors. Continued investment in medical research for chronic diseases and the processes of ageing will go on influencing the range of possible endings. The now somewhat discredited concept of cryogenic preservation suggested the possibility of an 'interrupted' curve. Whereas now there is the theoretical possibility of more deliberate life extension stretching out the curve still further (Kirkwood 2000). Altering the trajectory life in this direction is likely to challenge intuitions still further particularly if the price of such longevity is the necessity of voluntary squaring-off.

This digression into axiological trajectories is not without its purpose, since such reflections help to throw into relief some of our intuitions about what constitutes a fitting end to a life, a good death. If we ask directly what constitutes a good death, then there are many influences, which tend towards a defence of the norm that a complete and coherent life is a life lived to the end of the tail. Not the least of these influences is religious thought. The Judaic tradition emphasizes the importance of trying to preserve life even to its end and Christian thinking has had a particular influence on the hospice and palliative care movement. Christians, and specifically those active in providing hospice and palliative care usually reject out of hand all forms of proactive 'squaring-off', assisted suicide, euthanasia and terminal sedation. A rejection based, not only on the sanctity of life, but for the intrinsic value of the dying experience itself (Sacred Congregation for the Doctrine of the Faith 1980). We can make sense of this position in secular terms by invoking the concept of coherence discussed earlier. There is a sense in which living life to its 'natural' end could be seen to render the whole coherent and complete. Let us stay with this intuition for the moment — a good life is a coherent and complete life, a life lived to its natural end. Defending this intuition seems to offer a means of grounding the argument that justifies preserving the moratorium on assisted death. In contrast, if the analysis of the good death gives prominence to its experiential aspects, then it could equally be argued that living a life to its 'bitter end', where this includes many 'bad' experiences, adds no value to a life and may even positively detract from the quality and coherence of a life. In this case, a 'better' death may be achieved by active human intervention.

Good life, good death: a complex challenge

The rights and wrongs of end-of-life decisions, where these include assisted dying, often involve the drawing of a contrast between a death dictated by the rights of the autonomous individual, on the one hand, and the ideal of the good death on the other. This reinforces the view that these different perspectives must be seen as points on the opposite ends of a moral spectrum. Yet if we consider only the abstract qualities of a good death then there is a great deal of symmetry between these two positions. The ethical difference between the two positions is that, what can be directly strived for, on the one hand, may only be approached by what comes to the individual through moral luck or by negative engineering.

The history of modern palliative care is premised upon a movement that advanced an objective view of the good death. It offered the vision of a better way of dying when dying people had seemingly been abandoned by mainstream medicine. Palliative care has maintained the belief that it still has a substantive good to offer even in secular and diverse modern cultures. The ethical implications of such a conception is that there are a set of values that ought to be advanced and, in principle, 'dictated' to the individual as a better way of living life to its end. At the opposite end of the scale is the view, born of the cult of the individual, that there can be no such conception since each individual defines their own good. The ethical implication of individualism is that the individual ought to be free to dictate the nature of their own good death. This characterization in terms of polar differences not only embodies different ethics, but different politics, since each embodies two quite different conceptions about how the good life ought to be lived.

Palliative care, seen as a positive good, faces the practical challenge of how it ought to be practised. To have one's good dictated by a professional elite is a form of paternalism that has long been rejected. So is palliative care left to avow an ideal, but practice a compromise? Contemporary palliative care offers some alternative accounts. One positive portrayal of the palliative care ideal is that it shows, rather than imposes the good death, but in doing so proves its value both in the good it achieves and by attacking the alternative of assisted dying. A second is to see palliative care not as offering a substantive good, but as conforming to an ethical convention of rights that can only be negatively defined and, hence, can only offer a negative conception of what palliative care does. The negative conception of the good death is the ideally *palliatized* death. The ideally *palliatized* death allows death to happen — 'intends neither to hasten or postpone death' (WHO 2002). Palliative care on this model is wedded to an ideal of the 'natural death' in which people die of an underlying condition, rather than by human intervention. With the belief in the value of natural death, there comes a normative requirement to *die* a natural death and this imposes restrictions on what the individual can request for themselves. So that the distinction between the natural and the engineered can be cleanly maintained, it also requires a certain construction of what legitimate medical interventions aim at. This often appears as an 'artifactually' drawn divide; by this I mean a divide that requires a great deal of crafted argument to sustain, as is the case, for example, in the denial that there is a moral parallel between the withdrawal of life-sustaining treatment and assisted dying (Randall 2005; Randall and Downie 2006). The ideally *palliatized* death therefore becomes itself not a natural, but a socially constructed, form of dying.

The advocates of the engineered death are also wedded to an ideal, that of the autonomous life, another idealized position that should, and during the course of this book will, be subject to criticism (Woods 2005). However, those who advance a view of the good death that allows a greater role for individual control are also advancing a socially constructed form of dying. Both approaches share this in common and through this offers the potential for drawing the poles much closer together.

The morally pragmatic way forward is to seek to elaborate the complementary and potentially compatible aspects of these seemingly entrenched opposites and in this chapter I have attempted to suggest some common ground. The conceptual approach taken in this chapter has explored the potential common ground between these perspectives, in terms of the parameters of the good death. The palliative care approach accepts the value of respecting personal autonomy, but palliative care is wedded to a particular account of what is implied by such a principle. Palliative care also holds in common with advocates of assisted dying that it is right and desirable to manipulate certain aspect of the dying process in order to achieve a better death, and that some of this control and manipulation should be dictated by the patient. Whether this shared ground is a step towards a future reconciliation between the two positions remains to be seen.

3 Palliative care: history and values

Introduction

In this chapter, I turn to an account of the history of contemporary palliative care from its origins in the early modern hospice movement to the most recent commentary upon palliative care philosophy. A chapter length treatment of this complex history will always have its limitations, but as far as possible I shall attempt to be true to both the detail and to the conceptual complexities. My purpose in tracing the history of palliative care is to expose the underlying principles and core values that have shaped and are still significantly shaping its ongoing development.

This chapter is based upon a simple thesis: that palliative care is the successor to the modern hospice movement. Given that the principles and values of the hospice movement were strongly influenced by the Christian vocation to care for the dying, then these principles and values have also exerted an influence. However, as palliative care has evolved to become a distinct health discipline and a medical speciality, those principles and values have come under increasing pressure from competing values, which can be variously seen as undermining, distorting or even strengthening the distinctiveness of palliative care.

One such narrative portrays the evolution from vocation to medical discipline as being accompanied by a shift from a stoical Christian ethos to a gradual alignment with the secular liberal ethics of western medicine. Some of the tensions within palliative care arise through the attempt to maintain a distinctive palliative care value in the face of this pressure. Some notable commentators have attempted to steer a course around, what they regard as the worst aspects of contemporary medical ethics, consumerism and the excesses of liberal autonomy and reassert or indeed redefine a philosophy of palliative care (Kearney 2000; Randall and Downie 2006). The belief in a distinctive palliative care value set is something that is openly acknowledged, if not always clearly, and articulated within palliative care. Janssens (2001), for example, reports that only 13 per cent of delegates at a

European Association of Palliative Care (EAPC) conference believed that palliative care entails a religious set of values, although 53 per cent reported that the values of palliative care were different to other health practises. In contrast Randall and Downie's most recent book *The Philosophy of Palliative Care* (2006) challenges the contemporary philosophy of palliative care as being too 'Hippocratic' in its *modus operandi*, unduly influenced by modern medicine's values and approaches yet they also reaffirm what are quite standard medical values and approaches. Randall and Downie's is a subtle and complex critique and something I shall return to at the end of this chapter.

In tracing the history of palliative care, I shall attempt to make explicit its underpinning values, drawing where possible on the work of its pioneers and key commentators. I shall conclude the chapter by outlining what I see as the central values of palliative care, and consider whether these are secular or theistic in nature. I shall also examine the claims to the distinctiveness of palliative care and, in doing so, identify potential tensions and compatibilities between these and some of the competing ethical values.

Meanings and origins

The fact that there was a particular time when the phrase 'palliative care' was first coined has led several commentators to dwell upon the etymology of the term 'palliative' (Clark and Seymour 1999). Hence, Cicely Saunders' (1993) discussion of the Latin etymology of the word 'palliative' from the word for 'cloak' *(pallium)* and from this the Latin verb *palliare:* 'to cloak' or 'to hide'. The term clearly has a history of pejorative use and several of Cicely Saunders early discussions of the management of terminal illness reflect a negative meaning consistent with this history (Clark 1998). Although Morris (1997) offers an alternative etymology from the Greek term for 'shield', a suggestion that perhaps reveals more about the need to give a positive 'spin' to the dying business than merely scholarly interest. This in itself is indicative of the acute awareness within the palliative care community of the need to attend to the meaning of words, to avoid the negative connotations of some terms and to define 'palliative care' through numerous iterations in order to make its meaning and intent clear.

Saunders, in her earlier writing, describes terminal care as the point where 'comfort rather than curative or even *palliative procedures'* becomes the most appropriate approach (Saunders 1966: 225). This and other similar comments suggest that in the early phase of her work Saunders regarded 'palliative procedures' as something distinct from the main purpose of terminal care. Saunders comments: 'care for the dying person should be directed no longer towards his cure, rehabilitation or even palliation but primarily at his comfort' (Saunders 1967: 385). This might be taken to imply, as Gracia (2002) suggests, that palliative care had a quite separate and distinct evolution to that of hospice care; I believe that this suggestion is mistaken.

It is widely acknowledged that Balfour Mount probably coined the term 'palliative care' in 1973 to describe his hospital-based initiative to provide terminal care at the Royal Victoria Hospital, Montreal (Hamilton 1995; Billings 1998). It was certainly useful to have an alternative term to 'hospice' in a culture where this term was regarded as having negative connotations. However, the fact that Mount had spent a sabbatical period at St Christopher's and his acknowledgement that the Montreal initiative was itself modelled on St Christopher's, suggests a much closer alliance with the early UK hospice movement (Mount 1997). So the suggestion that 'palliative care' was born of a separate parallel evolution to that of hospice care is too strong a claim in the light of the available evidence. This is not to deny that Mount's terminology, and the underpinning practice this describes, had an influence upon Cicely Saunders who soon accepted that the concept of 'palliative care' was inclusive of the central elements of terminal care, which she had been advocating for over a decade (Clark 1999a, 2002a).

However, as Gracia (2002) discusses, the opening of a palliative care unit within an acute hospital setting could be usefully compared to the development of other medical specialities such as oncology and intensive care. Gracia suggests that there is an important comparison between the concepts of intensive treatment and palliative care. In oncology, the concept of intensified treatment, which aimed to cure, was an already established principle at the time in which the term 'palliative care' was coined. Intensification was itself contrasted with palliative treatment, which by implication, was less 'intense,' did not carry the same risk of iatrogenesis and did not aim to cure. A more significant contrast is, however, also suggested by Gracia, between the burgeoning philosophy of 'intensive care' and palliative care, he comments:

At the very beginning it was thought that intensive care should be the final way for all diseased human beings, either critically or terminally ill. At the end all human beings are in a critical situation.

(Gracia 2002: 30)

However, intensive treatment of the critically ill, if applied universally to all critically ill individuals, would lead to the over-treatment of the dying; the very outcome that hospice care had evolved to avoid. This is a problem distinct from, but as equally inappropriate, as the under-treatment of the dying. Both were concerns to the pioneers of the hospice movement, (Saunders 1987b). Saunders, reflecting on the origins of the hospice movement, noted that it was necessary to take dying people out of hospitals so that values could move back in. With the establishment of a palliative care unit within a hospital the question was whether these values could be preserved? In attempting to influence the approach of mainstream medicine, it was perhaps inevitable that palliative care would itself be influenced by the active approaches employed in the parallel disciplines of oncology and intensive care. A point to which I shall return in later discussion.

Palliative care the early phase: the modern hospice

If we accept that palliative care is the successor of hospice care, then it makes sense to talk of the 'early' phase of palliative care as originating in the modern hospice movement. Hospices, of course, have a much older heritage and, in her foreword to the *Oxford Textbook of Palliative Medicine*, as elsewhere in her writings, Cicely Saunders remarks upon this Christian heritage (Saunders 1993). For Saunders, the idea of a hospice as a place that provided hospitality to strangers resonated with her knowledge of and experience in the early hospices, which offered care for the dying. Saunders acknowledges that the term 'hospice' has different and perhaps less acceptable connotations in different contexts, but she notes that the nineteenth century saw parallel development of homes for the dying in England, in Ireland under the Irish Sisters of Charity, in France under Jean Garnier, and in other countries. Saunders goes on to comment: 'Most of the early homes and hospices were Christian in origin, their workers believing that if they continued faithfully with the work to which they felt called, help would reach their patients from God who had Himself died and risen again' (Saunders 2005: xix).

Although these homes for the dying were probably the models for the first generation of modern hospices, it was not until the 1950s and 1960s that a renewed interest in the plight of the terminally ill was taken. Clark (1999b, 2002b) observes that the rise of palliative care was shaped by four particular drivers, the first was the move towards an evidence-based practice, the second was a conscious engagement with values in the care of the dying, particularly that of open awareness, the third was a move away from stoicism to the adoption of a more active approach to caring for the dying, and the fourth was the adoption of an holistic approach to care. All of these drivers, but the first and fourth in particular, have gained still further momentum with the advent of palliative medicine as a distinct medical speciality. However, the momentum in the early phase, certainly in the UK context, was due, in no small part, to the efforts of nurses. It was Cicely Saunders, writing as a nurse, who was one of the early pioneering voices. The early development of palliative care can therefore be seen as sitting between these 'twin' histories, as Gracia (2002) puts it, between 'a little history and a big history of medicine' and Cicely Saunders, in her role as nurse and doctor, straddled both.

Like Cicely Saunders, many nurses were disillusioned by the lack of care for dying people. Nurses who migrated to hospice work did so out of compassion. Hospice work was caring and that is what nurses do, the motivation was from 'conviction', rather than an explicit awareness of 'ethics' as such (Gracia 2002: 93). Caring was also associated with Christian duty, rather than a nursing philosophy of care, although this too began to emerge. Cicely Saunders, wrote a series of highly influential articles in the *Nursing Times*, eventually published as a supplement entitled *Care of the Dying* (Saunders 1960). In this work, Saunders addresses issues ranging from euthanasia, symptom control, psycho-social and spiritual care, showing in nascent form ideas that later became central to palliative care philosophy.

Central to Saunders' view and that of other early nurse theorists, such as Virginia Henderson (1960), is the concept of 'holistic care'. Holism is the view that the person is a complex physical, psycho-social and spiritual entity, therefore requiring all of these aspects to be cared for. Holistic care has come to characterize a distinctive nursing theme and is widely discussed in the literature (Woods 1998). The acknowledgement of the importance of the holistic approach has become an abiding, if at times problematic value within palliative care shared by the multiple disciplines working in the field. Problematic because what holism implies in terms of the kind of service palliative care ought to provide to patients is open to question. The problem with a philosophy of care that incorporates complex ideals such as holism is that there is a gap between the ideal, and what is practical, deliverable and reasonable. Randall and Downie (2006) have rightly turned their critical attention to such concepts from the perspective that a philosophy of palliative care must be able to underpin what is expected of the practice.

David Clark's annotated bibliography of Saunders writing up to 1967 (Clark 1998) reveals a leitmotif of values with overt reference to the Christian duty to treat suffering, the emphasis on the importance of a community or *place* of care, and frequent reference to the 'real work' of terminal care, allowing space and peace for individuals to come to terms with their own death. However, as I have argued elsewhere (Woods *et al.* 2001) one needs to exercise caution and distinguish Saunders' personal religious conviction, and the expression of this in her early writing, from what she envisaged as a philosophy and deliverable service of hospice care. Alongside her reflections on Christian duty is an acute awareness of the need to bring practical and rational approaches to bear on solving the problems of pain and distress. In this early phase of palliative care, the emphasis was on establishing a place, rather than a transferable philosophy of care. The 'place' was outside of mainstream healthcare, where the dying could be cared for with due attention to both the patient and their family's needs. Saunders emphasized the need for a special place or community for the dying, what she called 'a stopping place for pilgrims' (Saunders 1962, 1964, 1973). Hence, the hospice was closely identified with a distinct building and a community of carers called to do that work.

Other agencies were also at play, recognizing and responding to the needs of the dying. Philanthropic individuals, some of whom were inspired by personal family experiences, took the lead in establishing charitable organizations to support dying people. In the UK in particular the establishment of two major cancer charities was influential in shaping the developing services for the terminally ill. The National Society for Cancer Relief, now Macmillan Cancer Relief, founded in 1919, and the Marie Curie Memorial, now Marie Curie Cancer Care founded in 1948 brought both resources and publicity to the cause (Raven 1990).

The Marie Curie Memorial, in conjunction with the Queen's Institute of District Nursing, conducted one of the first needs assessments of people terminally ill with cancer, cared for at home (Joint National Cancer Survey 1952). The survey conducted by district nurses visiting patients in their own homes, gathered data ranging from basic demographics to details of wound dressing requirements and spiritual needs. The clear association of poor social conditions and poverty with the greatest need provided evidence that terminal care must provide both health and social support. The report was one of the first pieces of evidence identifying the needs of families who were acting as the main carers. The report notes particularly the need for nursing care during the night and was one of the first to recognize the range of needs and subsequent types of services that would be required to meet such needs. The idea that palliative care must work in partnership with informal carers is a factor that has prevailed into contemporary palliative care approaches (Woods 2001).

The Marie Curie Memorial responded to the report by purchasing a number of large buildings and nursing homes to provide terminal and respite care, and by establishing a day and night nursing service as adjuncts to the statutory services. These were pragmatic responses, but taken in tandem with the developing philosophy of hospice care, the approach of providing care regardless of the patient's location has continued to be a distinctive feature of palliative care (Boyd 1995). Through these different mechanisms, both the needs of the terminally ill and the shape of an appropriate caring service began to be defined.

It became increasingly clear that terminally ill people were vulnerable in two particular ways. As hospital patients, terminally ill people were vulnerable to inappropriate treatment, whereas both hospital patients and those cared for at home were vulnerable to neglect of their particular needs, particularly for pain and symptom control. In addition, the report by Hughes (1960) identified the absence of a policy approach to this range of problems, without which there could be little hope of galvanizing the resources needed to address them.

Hospices, in this early phase, were places that provided primarily nursing care for the dying. Medical interventions, as such, were limited to attempts to control pain and other symptoms by the methods and means ready to hand. This care could be characterized as *passive*, allowing nature to take its course in the best possible circumstances. Although Cicely Saunders notes that one of her earliest and influential experiences as a nurse was to witness the regular administration of oral opiates; an established practice in St Luke's hospice.

It is difficult to say whether there was an awareness of explicitly ethical concerns in the hospice movement up to this point. Medical ethics was not the industry it has now become and there was not the same attention paid to making ethics so explicit. The plight of the dying was seen more as a failure of compassion and humanity, rather than labelled as a moral wrong. As far as it is possible to discern from the contemporary commentators on the modern hospices, the main concerns were about the appropriateness of care, the under-treatment of symptoms and the lack of attention to the issues that mattered, social, spiritual and psychological care. However, specifically *moral* concerns were being raised within the wider context of medicine. The recognition that the potential for over-treatment, as well as the potential for under-treatment to the point of neglect, was specifically recognized as an ethical challenge in the light of burgeoning medical technology, such as life-support equipment and methods (Jonsen 1990). However, the ethical implications of the use, withdrawing and withholding of such technology were made most apparent in the context of end-of-life care, and the obligations and duties of doctors to patients in such circumstances.

Some of the earliest explicitly *medical* ethical reflection upon the moral obligations of health workers was influenced by arguments from Catholic moral theology. These arguments offer an analysis of withholding or withdrawing such technology in terms of the scope of moral obligation in health care. The analysis distinguishes between the obligation to provide *ordinary* means of treatment and the absence of obligation to provide *extraordinary* means, expressed in the following way:

> Ordinary means are all medicines, treatments, and operations, which offer a reasonable hope of benefit and which can be obtained and used without excessive expense, pain, or other inconvenience. Extra-ordinary means are all medicines, treatments, and operations, which cannot be obtained or used without excessive expense, pain or other inconvenience, or which if used, would not offer a reasonable hope of benefit.

(Kelly 1951: 550)

This argument forms one of the key sources of the concepts of appropriateness and proportionality that have since become central to debates about the scope and aim of palliative care. However, the most relevant part of the argument is not the ambiguous distinction between ordinary and extraordinary means, but rather the phrase 'reasonable hope of benefit', a notion central to Randall and Downie's analysis of palliative care ethics (Randall and Downie 1999).

Although at the time of the development of the early hospices these were not debates that were seen as relevant. The idea that ethical concerns of the application of new medical technology might equally apply to a philosophy of care for the dying probably seemed remote. Hospices, as places away from mainstream healthcare, avoided being drawn into the debate because such resources were not ready to hand. This, together with the acknowledged imminence of death of hospice patients, meant that such questions did not arise. Yet hospice care might easily be seen to represent the withholding of life-sustaining treatment by default and that such withholding might also be regarded as ethically contentious. These are debates that just a few decades later were regarded as issues to which palliative care must have a response.

I would suggest that the modern hospice approach was not premised upon an ethical analysis of obligation, but was rather a much more intuitive response to the needs of the dying, and couched most often in an unreflective Christian duty towards the suffering and dying. In this sense, one could argue that the hospice response was morally pragmatic in the sense that I described in chapter 1. Hospice care was about caring for the dying and, since death was inevitable for hospice patients, their care was concerned with letting nature take its course in the least distressing way possible. The appropriateness of hospice interventions was therefore more easily circumscribed since hospice care was entirely focused upon the 'tail-end' of the prognostic trajectory. It was therefore easier to rule out a whole swathe of medical interventions as not appropriate. However, one area where more active intervention was necessary and showed some early promise was the control of pain. Saunders describes the attempts taken by early hospices such as St Luke's to adopt a systematic approach to achieving pain relief, approaches which inspired her own practice and informed her early research (Saunders 1994/5). This migration towards more active means of intervention came to characterize the nature of palliative care as essentially *active* in nature. The move towards more active measures might also be seen as entailing greater risk and, indeed, anxieties were expressed about the potential risks of over-using opiates, both at this time and since. The risk/benefits analysis was to become one of the central ethical concerns in contemporary palliative care.

Saunders' advocacy of effective symptom relief by the scientific application of drugs should be seen in conjunction with the other measures

Saunders described. Writing in the *Nursing Times,* Saunders (1959) emphasizes that pain can also be treated by 'physical nursing care', and by understanding physical and mental worries (1959: 1032). These two approaches combined, capture the essence of Saunders holistic approach to terminal care, something that was to become a pillar of palliative care philosophy.

Palliative care the middle phase: from hospice to palliative care

The middle phase of palliative care is arguably the period following the establishment of St Christopher's hospice in 1967. It was at this purpose-built institution that Cicely Saunders began to evangelize the hospice philosophy of terminal care through her teaching and writing (Clark and Seymour 1999). St Christopher's, as a purpose-built hospice, was arguably the first modern hospice. St Christopher's not only provided patient care, it had an active research programme, and provided education and 'internships' for professionals and, hence, representing a significant influence on palliative care. Despite the establishment of the National Health Service (NHS), providing State provision of health care within the UK, there was little attention given to terminal care within the NHS and the mostly Christian-based, charitably-funded hospices filled the gap. It was not until almost a decade later that the NHS began to provide continuing care facilities at a time when other purpose-built facilities and services began to evolve in other parts of the world (Clark *et al.* 2002).

The transition from hospice to palliative care is marked by the recognition that the principles of hospice care did not require a special place — a hospice — but could be applied wherever there was a need. This change of emphasis, refocusing upon the principles, rather than the place, can be seen as another of the key shifts in how palliative care began to be conceptualized. The shift from place to context is parallelled in the later shift in the point at which palliative interventions are deemed appropriate in the illness trajectory. This can be characterized as a change of emphasis 'upstream' from the terminal phase to a point much earlier in the illness trajectory. The 'upstreaming' of palliative care has come to characterize contemporary palliative care, but has also incurred problems in the conceptualization and principal values of palliative care. Points to which we shall return.

While there is no doubt that pioneers like Saunders and the UK hospices were leading influences on emerging palliative care, the shift from hospice to palliative care was also influenced by other developments on the international scene. By the 1970s there was a co-evolution of facilities and services, and a reciprocal influence in thinking. (Clark 1999a) suggests that

Saunders probable first use of the term 'palliative care' as synonymous with hospice care was in her letter to the *Canadian Medical Association Journal* in 1977 (Mount 1997), in which she acknowledges Balfour Mount's palliative care initiative. Saunders comments that Mount's work demonstrates the transferability of hospice principles to other contexts. In addition to acknowledging the flexibility of the hospice approach this period also saw the filling out of the substance of those principles. During this period, a palliative care literature began to evolve, addressing such issues as multidisciplinary working, evidence-based palliative care practice and the central concepts of total pain and total care (Clark and Seymour 1999)

Mount's initiative of locating a palliative care facility within a hospital setting had other implications. A palliative care facility as a 'unit' within a hospital forced palliative care to have an interface with medicine that the hospice located outside of the health services did not. In the hospital, palliative care becomes one speciality amongst many, and is subject to the bureaucracy and routines of the hospital. Some of this might be viewed as an advance, with access to services, equipment and technology, as well as to other medical specialties. However, this also created practical, conceptual and specifically ethical issues for both palliative care and other medical disciplines. Practical difficulties included the question of which service has responsibility for the palliative patient and which services can be accessed by the palliative patient? Conceptual challenges also because it was necessary to ask when does palliative care begin and who are the candidate recipients? Specifically ethical issues because there became a need to address questions concerning the use of artificial nutrition and hydration, to develop policies on cardio-pulmonary resuscitation; issues that were not so pressing when palliative care was limited to terminal care within the hospice setting.

In the UK, whether by chance or by design, some of these issues have been circumvented by locating palliative care facilities within hospital grounds, close, but not integrated with the hospital, although it is also the case that palliative care teams are increasingly working within the acute care setting. The interface of palliative care with mainstream medicine can be seen as both an opportunity and a threat. There is clearly an opportunity for palliative care to 'evangelize' out, spreading the principles and philosophy of palliative care to the acute sector. The threat that comes with this proximity is that it allows other powers to 'colonize' it. It is perhaps with specific focus on the context of palliative care within the hospital setting, that greatest credence may be given to the observations made by commentators in the 1990s that palliative care was being marred by medicalization and bureaucratization (James and Field 1992; Biswas 1993).

Palliative care the late phase: post-palliative medicine

By 1987, following the recognition of Palliative Medicine as a medical speciality in the UK, there was a new international recognition of the discipline and its aspirations. 'Hospice' was a word that had become rendered unacceptable by the relativity of the cultural meaning of that term. Although the word has been retained in some contexts and is still used to describe specialist palliative care units within the UK.

The emphasis within palliative care at this time was more focused upon the transferable principles of care that could be used to manage the needs of terminally ill people wherever they happened to be. There was also a more subtle, but conscious effort to move the concept of palliative care forward, away from the passive and negative associations of hospices with terminal care. This conceptual change can be traced most clearly in the UK context because it is well documented.

Until 2004, the umbrella organization the National Council for Hospices and Specialist Palliative Care Services (NCHSPCS) represented the palliative care community of the UK. In 2004, with a new constitution and a new name, this organization became the National Council for Palliative Care (NCPC). Whether deleting the reference to hospices in the organization's title has any symbolic, rather than practical significance is open to debate. There is no doubt that the word was not regarded as entirely neutral, and its association with death might be seen to have a negative effect on a new and dynamic health discipline.

The move towards defining and advancing a philosophy of palliative care has been a deliberate and active one. The NCHSPCS (1995) *A Statement of Definitions* was the product of a members' working party consensus on key definitions. This attempt at defining key concepts begins to distinguish hospice and palliative care, as well as mapping out distinctions within palliative care itself. Key distinctions are drawn between palliative care in general, the palliative care approach, and specialist palliative care (NCHSPCS 1995). One of the factors behind this taxonomical exercise is specific to the UK and the NHS. It is an attempt to clarify the nature of palliative care for potential commissioners of palliative care services. One interpretation of this repackaging exercise is that it provided a means of strengthening the position of palliative care services by securing central resources. A second, more speculative factor is ideological in that by defining and redefining key concepts the role of palliative medicine as central to the discipline is confirmed. However, it should also be acknowledged that the need to establish a consensus around the definitions and key goals of palliative care was something that was being addressed at the international level. Palliative care was being presented as something *active* and not about a stoical acceptance of death. The World Health Organization's (WHO) definition of palliative care as: 'The active total care of patients whose disease is not responsive to curative treatment' (WHO 1990: 11) was being echoed in the various national and international consensus statements that have become such a feature of contemporary palliative care (ten Have and Clarke 2002).

The NCHSPCS document should also be seen in the context of appearing towards the end of the first decade of palliative medicine as a recognized medical speciality when there was perhaps a stronger feeling of self-assurance within the discipline. The document also coincides with yet another round of NHS reforms in which positioning for funding was crucial. The document begins by defining palliative care with the familiar list of values and goals:

> Palliative care is the active total care of patients and their families by a multi-professional team when the patient's disease is no longer responsive to curative treatment.
>
> (NCHSPCS 1995: 5)

Hospice care is, however, described as a 'philosophy of care', but one that does not define the 'range and quality of the service' as, by implication, this document purports to do for palliative care. The document can be read in two ways, as an attempt to demarcate and define a specialist service to potential purchasers and, given the singular reference to hospice care, and the now change of name of the NCHSPCS to the National Council for Palliative Care, expunging an historical association that has been outgrown.

Describing hospice care as a 'philosophy' renders it necessarily vague and, hence, less useful in selling a health service to purchasers. A further consideration is the historical association of hospices exclusively with *terminal* care. Although the NCHSPCS statement acknowledges terminal care as an important part of palliative care, it is applicable only during the last few weeks or months of life. Terminally ill people are defined as those individuals who can reasonably be expected to die within 12 months (NCHSPCS 1995: 5). The subsuming of terminal care within palliative care could be seen as a means of extending the scope of palliative care and is indicative of the 'upstreaming' approach that was a distinctive feature of palliative care during the 1990s.

The agenda of setting the widest possible frame of reference for palliative care could also be seen as evidence of the process of medicalization. The earlier within the disease trajectory that palliative care is deemed appropriate then the wider the scope there is for palliative medicine to intervene. The reduced emphasis upon terminal care may also be seen as a sign of a profession uncomfortable with the concept of 'incurability' and the explicit spiritual goals of the hospice movement in particular. However, one must be cautious not to read too much into either the concept or the process of medicalization as applied to palliative care. Clark and Seymour (1999) observe that the medicalization thesis began as a sociological observation and critique of an increasingly powerful medical profession, which began to exert its influence upon post-war society. Medicine was a profession with strong scientific credentials, a rational agenda and with legitimate claims to efficacy, which bolstered its authority. Later commentators saw the process and effects of medicalization in more pejorative terms. James and Field (1992), for example, in the vein of Illich (1976), see the encroaching medicalization of palliative care as part of an expanding domain of social control, avoiding talk of death by emphasizing chronic disease, failing to engage with the requirements of the holistic approach by focusing upon the control of symptoms. Biswas (1993) expressed concerns of a different kind, that medicalization represents the displacement of nursing as the lead discipline in terminal care. However, such charges must be balanced against the successes that medicine has achieved in underpinning successful symptom control with scientific knowledge and converting an *ad hoc* charity-based alliance into a recognized health discipline increasingly underpinned with central resources. Nor must it be forgotten that Cicely Saunders herself became a doctor in order to become more efficacious in dealing with the challenges of terminal illness. Saunders' approach seems to combine the best of a medical scientific approach with a compassionate humanity.

While there are some differences in ideology and values between hospice care and palliative care, which are, in part, due to medicalization there is also much continuity. An abiding aspect of both hospice and palliative care is the need to engage in the explicit articulation of a philosophy and set of values that is unique within a health discipline. What has also continued is the task of providing a rational basis for care, and, in so far as medicine has generally sought a strong evidence base, this is one area where medical influence has been greatest. A further area of continuity is the emphasis placed upon the respect owed to the dying person up to the point of death, and that the task of providing the requisite care necessitates the expertise of a number of professions and, hence, the recognition of the multi-disciplinary team approach in which nursing remains a core discipline. Palliative care has also continued the tradition of adopting a strong stance against euthanasia. If there is less emphasis upon terminal care then this is perhaps because of the increased ability to recognize incurable illness at a point in time well in advance of the terminal stages of a disease. In a sense, this is indicative of the Janus like nature of palliative care with its two faces pointing in opposite directions. One face turned upstream towards chronic disease, and the other towards the terminal phase and death. In her introduction to the *Oxford Textbook of Palliative Medicine* (2005) Cicely Saunders manages to paint a coherent picture of palliative care which conceals such tensions. She states:

All the work of the professional team — the increasingly skilled symptom control, the supportive nursing, the social and pastoral work, the home care and the mobilization of community resources enable people to live until they die ... Patients should end their lives in the place most appropriate to them and to their families, and where possible have choice in the matter. Some insight into the serious nature of their disease by the patient will help towards realistic decisions ... When a person is dying the family find themselves in a crisis situation, with the joys and regrets of the past, the demands of the present, and the fears of the future, all brought into stark focus. Help may be needed to deal with guilt depression and family discord, and in this time of crisis there is the possibility of dealing with old problems and finding reconciliations that greatly strengthen the family. If this time is to be used there needs to be some degree of shared awareness of the true situation. Truth needs to be available (though not pressured) so that the family can travel together ... The often-surprising potential for personal and family growth at this stage is one of the strongest objections most hospice workers raise for the legalization of a deliberately hastened death or for an automatic policy of 'shielding' the patient from the truth ... Now that palliative care is spreading worldwide it has still, according to the definition of the World Health Organization kept a concern for the spiritual needs of its patients and their families. The whole approach has been based on the understanding that a person is an indivisible entity, a physical and spiritual being.

(Saunders 2005: xix)

In these few eloquent paragraphs, Saunders distils the basic tenets of palliative care in a way that dismisses many of the potential tensions I have begun to identify. Although the WHO definition has since altered in emphasis from the 1990 version cited by Saunders in this passage. The more recent WHO definition of palliative care states:

Palliative care is an approach that improves the quality of life of patients and their families facing the problems associated with life-threatening illness, through the prevention and relief of suffering by means of early identification and impeccable assessment and treatment of pain and other problems, physical, psycho-social and spiritual.

(WHO 2002)

This definition of palliative care, although seemingly consistent with some of the aspirations of palliative I have been exploring in this chapter, is seen by some as vague and potentially damaging. In describing palliative care as an approach the WHO definition has failed to reinforce the distinctiveness of the expertise which palliative medicine regards as central to the speciality. Also by giving prominence to the quality of life goals of palliative care something of the more concrete goals and aims are lost. So *when* ought palliative care be offered and to *whom* remains a legitimate question? These are criticisms to which I shall return.

Contemporary palliative care in the UK

Saunders summary of palliative care can be summarized still further into a list of the central components of palliative care:

- Scientifically robust treatment of symptoms.
- Team approach to care provision.
- Choice in place of dying.
- Open awareness with patient and family.
- Psychological care of patient and family.
- Belief in the potential for growth.
- Opposition to assisted dying.
- Holistic approach to the person.

This bulleted summary of the principles and values of palliative care has become an increasingly strong mantra from the time of the founding of St Joseph's hospice in 1967 yet it has taken almost four decades for this to have an impact on policy. Seymour (2001) has catalogued the continuing failure of medicine to deal humanely with dying people, this work adding to the established and growing body of work with the same litany of complaints that inspired the first hospices. So, although the palliative care community seems to know what it ought to be doing there has been a problem in translating this into practice.

Most of this chapter has focused upon the situation in the UK, partly because it is home to so many pioneers and partly because the history is so well documented. However, even in the UK, said to have one of the most advanced palliative care services in the world, the advances in applying a comprehensive palliative care service have been modest and piecemeal.

It is curious that the problems encountered by dying people and their families and the strategies to deal with them were extensively described in the 1950s (Joint National Cancer Survey 1952; Hughes 1960). However, things are seemingly set to change following a series of policy initiatives and reforms over the past decade. The so called 'Calman/Hine' Report [Department of Health/Welsh Office (DOH/WO) 1995], which established a framework for cancer services across England and Wales was one of the first strategies to give impetus to palliative care, and its integration with cancer services. Further impetus was given by the NHS Cancer Plan (2000), which promised to increase the standard of care for the dying. More recently, a range of strategies to plan for end of life care have been implemented in the form of the NHS end-of-life care programme and the creation of National Services Frameworks, which have incorporated aims for appropriate end-of-life care across other chronic diseases and for older people. The NHS Confederation published a summary of Government and wider agency responses to the challenge of improving end-of-life care (NHS 2005). The approach outlined in this summary goes a long way to reconciling some of the tensions that have existed between hospitals and palliative care, between terminal care and palliative medicine, and between cancer and other chronic incurable conditions. It is acknowledged that end-of-life care is part of a much wider area of palliative care and that there is a need to galvanize services and resources across the health and social sectors to meet the increasing needs of an ageing population. What is significant about the response is that it incorporates many of the principles and values of palliative care into professional standards, guidelines and protocols (Ellershaw 2002; Ellershaw and Wilkinson 2003; Thomas 2003) The programme is also underwritten by government funding including incentives to general practitioners to specialise in end-of-life care (General Medical Services Contract 2004). The Gold Standards Framework (GSF) for community palliative care (Thomas 2003) was developed to provide a framework for primary care professionals to manage patients in their last year of life. The GSF enables support to be given to patients and their carers, access to specialist palliative care, avoids emergency admission and respects the patient's choice of place of death. The Liverpool Care Pathway, LCP, (Ellershaw and Wilkinson 2003) helps generalist staff to provide terminal care in hospital in the last 48 hours of life, and seems to be taking back into hospitals the skills and values that necessitated patients' removal to hospices four decades earlier. The overall thrust of the programme is impressive, seeming to incorporate many of the ideals of palliative care. Practical meaning is given to the difference between specialist palliative care and the palliative care approach, the multi-disciplinary team is seen as central, diseases other than cancer are recognized and death as a social reality is acknowledged. Particular emphasis is given to consumerism and patient choice, what might be labelled as patient 'autonomy', with regard to choice of place of death and advance planning including advance choice about treatment and care options making use of the legal recognition of advance directives. So has the palliative care ideal been realized? The end-of-life care programme is still in its infancy and its impact must wait to be seen. There are, of course, further challenges of a conceptual and ethical in nature, and I now turn to these.

Conceptual and ethical issues

In mapping the development of palliative care three stages have been described. The earliest stage of development takes as its focus a concern with terminal care, and with the establishment of a place or sanctuary for the dying. The middle period of development is co-extensive with the development of the modern hospice movement. Although this period continued to share the earlier preoccupation with the provision of terminal care within a hospice, it was also shaped by a growing recognition of the need for flexibility in the provision of hospice care. In addition to providing good physical care combined with psycho-social and spiritual aspects of dying for both patient and their family there was a growing emphasis on scientifically-based symptom control. The contemporary and still evolving phase is that of palliative care proper, which includes both specialist palliative care and the palliative care approach. The palliative care approach is an overarching *philosophy* of care (NCHSPCS 1995: 5), incorporating the basic principles of palliative care to be employed across the spectrum of health care. Specialist palliative, according to the same source of definitions, is delivered by a specifically trained multi-professional team dealing with complex pain and other symptoms, working either directly with the patient wherever they may be or by advising an intermediary professional. The LCP is a very successful example of how specialist palliative care has supported the application of the palliative care approach in the hospital setting (Ellershaw 2002). However, a narrower interpretation of specialist palliative care might see palliative care as a strategy for the advancement of a particular form of medical speciality, palliative medicine.

The broad international consensus regarding the aims of palliative care revolves around the World Health Organization's definition of palliative care. That is not to say that within the palliative care community there are no dissenters with regard to the scope and demarcation of palliative care. I have described the development of palliative care within the UK as an exemplar and one of the major influences upon palliative care, but the UK is also complicated by its history of charitable and State funded provision of health care running in parallel; something that will also continue even under the new programme for end-of-life care.

Even though it could be said to be now accepted that palliative care is not just for cancer, a problem remains. The aspiration to 'upstream' palliative care now means that there is a puzzle as to who palliative care is for and which interventions are appropriate. Some commentators continue to be dissatisfied with the absorption of terminal care, the main purpose of hospices, into palliative care, fearing that this aspect will be lost in a service focused upon 'acute' outcomes (Biswas 1993). The aspiration to widen the scope of palliative care to all 'active progressive disease' is limited by the fact that much of the expertise within palliative care is related to advanced cancer and in the UK particularly this aspiration runs counter to the vested interests of the powerful cancer charities who play a crucial role in the provision of palliative care services; although the central funding of the new programme may go some way to resolving this matter.

Funding palliative care is also a global issue since the placing of palliative care within mainstream medical services means that palliative care is competing for resources with other services. So how palliative care is defined in terms of its scope and application might be seen as crucial for its success in this competition. The WHO definition talks only of an 'approach' and fails to emphasize the existence of and need for a distinct speciality. A second issue is the scope of the commitment; something that Randall and Downie (2006) regard as a significant challenge. In their critique of the philosophy of palliative care they regard the values implicit within the WHO philosophy as over-committing palliative care services in a way that entails unethical macroallocation of resources. They argue specifically that, in addition to the assessment and treatment of the patient's symptoms, palliative care is obliged to assess, monitor and treat the psychosocial, spiritual and quality of life needs of both the patient and their family. This, they argue, requires more of palliative care than any other health speciality. Randall and Downie have specific concerns both regarding the detail of what the philosophy of palliative care commits the service to and to the possible volume of demand. In particular, they argue that because the philosophy does not discriminate between a need and a capacity to benefit, palliative care is obliged to attempt to meet what is potentially an infinite demand. As a specific commentary that demands particular attention, I shall return to Randall and Downie's critique at the end of this chapter. First, I shall offer my own analysis of some of the challenges represented by attempts since the 1990s to develop and operationalize palliative care philosophy.

The WHO definition of palliative care emphasizes the overlap with curative interventions such as cancer therapies. This is vague in a number of ways as it makes it difficult to characterize who is responsible for palliative care, when it is appropriate, and what distinct contribution palliative care makes. Hence, the NCHSPCS (1995) attempt to make the distinction between the approach and the speciality clear. Specialist palliative care is a multi-disciplinary approach with a high level of training to deal with complex symptoms, such as refractory pain, dyspnoea and agitation, and is capable of delivering such care wherever the patient may be. However, the distinction between the approach and the specialist work of palliative care may be clear enough at one level of analysis, but far from clear when attempting to identify either the general goals of palliative care or the appropriateness of specific treatments and interventions. Because palliative care purports to embrace the upstream phase of care the context is more complex than if it were limited to the terminal phase alone. What might be reasonable to expect a patient to suffer in terms of inconvenience, risk and side effects must be balanced against the fact that the palliative patient cannot be cured and has a limited life span. For this reason, the terms reasonableness, proportionality and appropriateness are commonly used in an attempt to express the kind of judgement upon which interventions rest. These concepts are inherently vague because their meaning is relative and contextual, but as discussed in chapter 2, they are premised upon plausible intuitions. However, these intuitions become less plausible the further upstream that palliative care intervention is applied because the further away the patient is from the terminal phase of their condition.

In the palliative context commentators often refer to the challenge of determining the status of the patient on the illness trajectory; from the potentially curable to the terminally ill. Conceptualizing such trajectories are proving useful in anticipating needs over time leading up to death (Lynn and Adamson 2003). It has been suggested that typical illness trajectories may provide a useful tool for addressing such common questions such as 'how long have I got?' and 'What will happen?' Being able to respond to such questions with reasonably predictive, if general, data would prove invaluable for planning services. Indeed, a strength of the UK's end-of-life programme is that such trajectories are being utilized, both to inform service planning and to enhance patient and family autonomy; enabling them to prepare for future events.

The intention of palliative care to move beyond the cancer model to address the needs of people with a range of chronic diseases is also a particular challenge. Palliative care aspires to be applicable early in the disease process, however, because there is no single trajectory for advancing chronic disease, this presents a specific challenge to the evolving model of palliative care. The aspiration to move away from this model may yet prove over-reaching, making it difficult for palliative medicine in particular to maintain the identity of a medical speciality. However, it is the specifically ethical implications for the proportionality and appropriateness of interventions that I wish to discuss here.

Perhaps the earliest and most simplistic model for the relationship between curative and palliative care is a straightforward linear model as represented in Figure 3.1.

The problem with this model is its simplistic separation of the curative

Figure 3.1

Diagnosis	Curative treatment	Palliative treatment	Terminal care	Death

from the palliative phases of care. On this model, all attempts to cure the disease are appropriate and, hence, proportionate up to the mysterious point of transition from curative to palliative. It fails to recognize that chronic and progressive disease may have an impact much earlier in the disease trajectory, and it has implications for both the type of service and place in which care is provided. This model's inadequacy is consistent with a medical model that is overly optimistic with respect to the application of medical technologies, regards death as a failure, and is least likely to engage in an open and honest discussion with the patient and family. It is also, however, a model to which patients and their families may also subscribe, having high expectations of contemporary medicine (Murray *et al.* 2005). Paradoxically, this model seems also to be compatible with the modern hospice approach where the privileged terminally ill are 'rescued' from the failures of mainstream healthcare and sequestrated in a special place until their death. Even if such a system were made sustainable by increasing the number of hospices it seems unrealistic on a number of fronts. The shift from curable to terminal is neither a discrete event nor is there a single trajectory against which to plot a patient's decline. Moreover, the approach is incongruous both with the range of patient's wishes and with the aspiration that medicine ought to be able to deal with both cure and death.

An early attempt to utilize a more complex and subtle trajectory model can be seen in the analysis offered by Ashby and Stoffell (1991). Although this model has echoes of the linear approach, Ashby and Stoffell argue that it is important to establish the status of the patient on the illness trajectory in order to justify the 'therapeutic ratio', the relationship between the invasiveness of treatment balanced against its burden to the patient. This relationship can be described in terms of an inverted wedge model (Figure 3.2).

Figure 3.2   The inverted wedge model

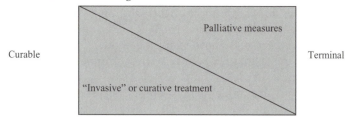

The intuition on which this model is premised is that as a person's disease progresses from a potentially curable condition to a no longer curable condition over a predictable period of decline in which there is a justifiable change in emphasis of treatment and care. During this transition the sort of treatment that is appropriate can be expressed in terms of the ratio between what is proportionate, and what is too invasive or burdensome. Over the course of this trajectory, treatment will alter in favour of palliative and less burdensome interventions carrying lower risk of treatment related morbidity and mortality. However, judging the appropriateness of an intervention and gauging the shift in the therapeutic ratio is complex and, at times, controversial. For example, who is to judge the meaning of 'burdensome', which may be described conceptually as 'disproportionate' to a particular goal, but may, from a patient's own perspective, be tolerable and desirable.

Yet, to do justice to the context of end-of-life decisions, there is a necessity to engage with this complexity. The inverted wedge model demonstrates quite clearly the concept of the 'upstreaming' of palliative care, suggesting that palliative care can begin very early in the disease trajectory so long as palliative care is understood in terms, not of terminal care, but quality of life goals.

However, some of the most challenging ethical problems arise over disputes about what is and is not appropriate throughout this trajectory. These disputes are not only fuelled by doctors unfamiliar with palliative care and unwilling to accept death, but by patients and their families (Slevin *et al.* 1990; Boyd 2002; Evans 2004; Gostin 2005). There is a need to be more specific about what is and what is not appropriate by at least elaborating the grounds on which these sorts of decision are made. There is some consensus among palliative care professionals, at least with respect to the phase when death is imminent. Some interventions seem to be definitively ruled out, as Ellershaw and Ward (2003) discuss in what might be described as the 'new terminal care':

> Non-essential drugs should be discontinued. Drugs that need to be continued, such as opioids, anxiolytics, and anti-emetics should be converted to the subcutaneous route ... Inappropriate interventions, including blood tests and measurement of vital signs, should be discontinued. Evidence is limited but suggests that continuing artificial fluids in the dying patient is of limited benefit and should in most cases be discontinued. Patients who are in the dying phase should not be subject to 'cardiopulmonary resuscitation', as this constitutes a futile and inappropriate medical treatment.
>
> (Ellershaw and Ward 2003: 32)

This is plain and robust advice in a context that seems unambiguous. This approach is perhaps indicative of the potential the LCP has to influence terminal care in the non-specialist settings. However, judging the appropriateness of an intervention and gauging the shift in the therapeutic ratio is complex and, at times, controversial (Gillick 2005). Ellershaw and Ward themselves acknowledge the difficulty in diagnosing dying, which is limited, in their words, to when the patient has 'only hours or days to live'

(2003: 31), but this represents only the final tip of the palliative care 'wedge'.

What Ellershaw and Ward describe as appropriate in the final hours and days is therefore not really 'new terminal care', but rather traditional hospice care imported with some confidence into a non-hospice setting. However, the establishment of palliative medicine as a medical speciality has, in contrast, been attended by a willingness to use more 'medical' and 'invasive' interventions and, because it aspires to reach earlier into the disease trajectory, must encounter territory where the picture is not so clear. As I argued in chapter 2 that the appropriateness of care is dependent upon the clarity of the goals of care and the upstreaming of palliative care means that these goals become more difficult to define.

The upstreaming of palliative care combined with the broadening of its involvement to diseases, other than cancer, adds another layer of complexity because, for example, the illness trajectories of heart failure, neuromuscular conditions and dementia do not follow the predictable pattern of incurable cancer (Murray *et al.* 2005). With other conditions, such as HIV/AIDS and the haematological malignancies it is even more difficult to judge appropriateness because even palliative measures can be very invasive and burdensome; in these circumstances there may be even greater scope for the patient to determine what is and is not appropriate (Robert and Solomon 2005).

One solution lies within palliative care, and its commitment to open awareness and good communication. Ideally, the gradual transition through the illness trajectory, and the adjustments in treatment this necessitates, can be negotiated between patient and doctor in a context in which greater priority is given to the patient's views. This approach is consistent with both contemporary approaches with respect for patient autonomy, and with a presumption that patients have an insight into their own quality of life that takes priority over the views of others at least in terms of their right to refuse treatment; an area of complexity and controversy to which we shall return.

The fact that many 'palliative' patients are cared for in the acute setting raises specific ethical issues of cardio pulmonary resuscitation (CPR), the use of life sustaining treatment, involvement in clinical trials and quality of care. The fact that there is a presumption in favour of CPR in acute hospitals emphasizes the importance of and need for a clear policy coupled with effective communication. Yet some patients are reluctant to have such a conversation, as are some doctors to initiate it, some patients are shocked to hear that they are not being considered for resuscitation and others, when communication fails, are subject to futile attempts (Conroy *et al.* 2006).

However, even to accept the position advanced by Ellershaw and Ward (2003) raises problems for concepts like futility. Futility is not a diagnosis

as such, but a value judgement and there have been suggestions that '...
futility judgements allow the doctors and the courts to camouflage conflicts
of value with the respectability of a valid clinical decision' (Maclean
2001: 784). This comment has a particular resonance when one considers
that '... [t]here is much disagreement about the meaning of medical futility
... Futility means different things to different people, who then argue with
one another as if they were talking about the same thing' (Taylor and
Lantos 1995: 3)

An additional complication is that of determining exactly what constitutes a 'burden' and from whose perspective the weight of such a burden
is judged. This is perhaps borne out by Slevin *et al.*'s study (1990), which
showed that people with advanced cancer are willing to carry a greater risk
of morbidity and mortality in the hope of a remission than are doctors,
nurses and matched members of the public. This perhaps suggests that
treatment cannot be too *aggressive* if it is at the patient's request, but such a
claim is at odds with some of the central tenets of palliative care that would
regard refusing such requests as imposing justified limits upon autonomy.

So the several attempts by palliative care professionals to make sense of
the concepts of the *appropriateness* of interventions in terms of *burden-
someness* and *proportionality* of treatment remain questionable over and
above the inherent ambiguity of these terms. Perhaps the biggest challenge
is that of *whose* interpretation should be given priority?

A specific challenge for the Ashby and Stoffell (1991) model is their
presumption in favour of a smooth linear progression from the curable to
incurable and from the appropriateness of burdensome interventions to
these becoming disproportionate. Ahmedzai (1996) offers his own critique
of linear models, arguing that there is no discernible point of transition
from curative to palliative care, and from palliative to terminal care. In
describing the 'Sheffield' model of palliative care, Ahmedzai likens the
process from diagnosis to death as more of an analogue than a digital
progression, with palliative care overarching the full progress with an
emphasis on *quality* of life goals, rather than *quantity* of life goals (Clark
and Seymour 1999: 85). Ahmedzai's approach is, however, complicated by
a potential conflict with other attempts to define palliative care and
demarcate palliative care from specialist palliative care, and specialist
palliative care from other specialisms. However, in Ahmedzai's account it is
not clear which interventions count as palliative care and which as acute
care, unless it is by reference to the 'specialist' who provides the intervention and, hence, circularity is introduced into the meaning.

It is also contentious to claim that attention to psycho-social, spiritual
and family needs, are distinctive of the '*palliative* care approach' since these
are the non-disease related goals, which are central to nursing models of
care. This may be to misconstrue Ahmedzai's point, which clearly says
something important about the nature of palliative care, but fails to satisfy

all of the relevant conceptual issues. Ahmedzai does make a good case for the upstreaming of palliative care, but a case that runs the risk of undermining the very coherence of palliative care as something distinct. This may not be a problem, but rather the case of palliative care taking its place among the other medical disciplines. However, if this is the case then it becomes more problematic to claim that palliative care has a distinct axiology or value set from that of secular liberal medical ethics.

This brings me finally to Randall and Downie's critique of palliative care philosophy (Randall and Downie 2006), which represents both a challenge to liberal medical ethics and offers a potential alternative in the form of the Asklepian model.

My first observation is that the *The Philosophy of Palliative Care* (2006) offers little new in substance from the arguments developed in their earlier *Palliative Care Ethics* (Randall and Downie 1999). The main difference between the two books is that their most recent volume sets out to offer a critique, in the sense of a systematic evaluation of strengths and weaknesses, of the philosophy of palliative care implicit in the WHO (2002) definition. In addition, they propose, with all due modesty and caution, their own alternative. I do not propose to conduct a detailed analysis of this book; I would encourage readers to do this for themselves. I will, however, pick out a number of the salient arguments and conclusions, referring in more detail to these in subsequent chapters.

In the first part of their book, Randall and Downie consider the form of the WHO statement and whether it does in fact constitute a philosophy. They conclude that since it functions as a normative statement of beliefs intended to influence practice then it does represent a kind of philosophy, but akin to an ideology. The WHO statement offers no reasoned arguments, but Randall and Downie argue that these can be unpacked by examining the trends in practice the beliefs encourage. The distinction drawn between a philosophy and an ideology is well made, and the authors are appropriately cautious about their own offering. They do, in fact, develop their own reasoned arguments in the context of the critique they make of the standard practises in palliative care of which they disapprove.

There is a three-fold aim to the book: to show how palliative care has strayed from its ideals and values, to revive the original ideals and values, and to steer practice towards betterment. In establishing the basis of their critique, Randall and Downie note, in passing, the Christian Heritage that informed and inspired the early hospices. However, they move on to locate the contrast between the hospice approach, its acceptance of mortality and attention to holistic care, and the aggressive pursuit of a cure by mainstream medicine, as rooted in a much older tradition. This older tradition derives from the two great healers of antiquity, Hippocrates and Asklepius. Hippocrates inspired the Hippocratic approach of rational scientific medicine, which focused on understanding disease and curing it. The Asklepian tradition, as Kearney (2000) describes in his earlier account of its relevance to palliative care, accepts human mortality and focuses upon healing, rather than cure. The tradition recognizes that people need space and peace in order to allow healing from the inside. Randall and Downie liken the Asklepian doctor's practice to the gaze of the harmless snakes who inhabited the temples of Asklepius, attending to the patient with their gaze, but not intruding. As an heuristic device, this analogy works to the extent that it enables Randall and Downie to make the charge that traditional 'Asklepian' palliative care has become infected by Hippocratic approaches. The main symptoms of this infection are hidden by the rhetoric of holistic care, and attention to spiritual and psycho-social needs, which has become the host to intrusive measurement and assessment tools, and intrusive interventions imposed upon the patient without their consent. Their conclusion, which is well argued for, is summarized in their own philosophy statement. In this statement, they try to capture the balance between Hippocratic and Asklepian virtues dealing, with patients' need for good symptom control in a consensual and fair way. They askew responsibility for treating the family of the patient, and restrict responsibility to treating what palliative care can diagnose and treat without taking responsibility for the sum of a person's problems. The new philosophy is modest, reasonable and humane, although I shall examine some of the detail of these arguments in subsequent chapters. At first glance some of the changes the authors propose, for example the emphasis on consent, the exclusivity of doctor/patient relationships, a costs/benefits model for decision-making, sound like a restatement of some traditional medical values. This is significant because one of the early motives in the founding of the modern hospice movement was the fact that medicine had failed the dying! This same claim remains significant in current critical commentary with concerns expressed that the medicalization of palliative care is once again failing the dying. On my analysis the philosophy of palliative care is really a philosophy of palliative medicine.

Conclusion

This chapter has outlined the key stages of development in palliative care, as well as defining some of the concepts and terms that help to both define and demarcate palliative care from the rest of medicine. The rich and complex history of palliative care in the UK means that both the range of issues and the breadth of scholarship dealing with those issues are considerable. Inevitably, more than a summary consideration of these issues has been impossible here; however, I have tried to identify the strengths of the emerging discipline, as well as identify some of the weaknesses in the conceptual analysis of palliative care and its goals. To emphasize palliative care as an adjunct to medicine, even if this is to emphasize the wider goals than cure, is to rob palliative care of something distinctive and, indeed, identity constituting. The ideals of the early hospice movement focused upon the possibility of the good death and enabling natural death to become the good death through proper care and symptom control.

Palliative medicine is now a well established sub-speciality of medicine and the whole range of health professional groups are involved in palliative care delivery. Yet despite the aspiration to apply palliative care to all chronic progressive diseases, it has remained a service mostly directed towards people with cancer (Higginson 1997; National Council for Hospice and Specialist Palliative Care Services 1998), although the UK's end-of-life programme aspires to change this pattern and make palliative care for all a reality (Clark 2006).

The willingness to shift the focus of palliative care upsteam has meant there are now more ethical issues to be faced than fewer. In the following chapters, I shall articulate what I regard as the distinctive palliative care value framework and apply this to some of the ethical challenges.

4 Ethics in palliative care: autonomy and respect for persons

Introduction

One of the questions I have been exploring in this book is whether there is a philosophy of palliative care and a distinct set of values to accompany it? I am interested in identifying those principles and values, observing their evolution over time and examining their adequacy as a context for contemporary death and dying. In chapter 2, I examined some intuitions about the nature of the good death. I concluded that, although the good death may seem highly individual, it is nested within broader concepts of the good life in which there are many parameters held in common.

I am also interested in examining the constraints and opportunities there are for individuals to shape their own good death. I suggest that a good philosophy of palliative care is able, not only, to justify the constraints and opportunities it advocates, but to have a view as to why *this* way is better. To conduct this analysis, it is necessary to engage in some theory. In particular, it is necessary to unpick some ethical concepts such as autonomy and respect for persons that seem central to this discussion. It will be recalled that in chapter 2 I argued for a pragmatic approach to ethics. I also made the particular point that 'ethics' understood as a moral practice is not driven by theory. So why indulge in a theoretical discussion now? For two reasons — the first is that theory is useful for identifying contexts and for unpicking and analysing arguments. The second is that some level of theory is necessary when generating new arguments. I made the point in chapter 2 that ethics is not just about habits and practises, but requires a degree of reflexivity in order to scrutinize the adequacy of those habits and practises. Randall and Downie's *The Philosophy of Palliative Care* (2006) is a good example of a pragmatic approach. Randall and Downie are critical of too much theory, and they locate the ethics and values of palliative within its practises. However, in offering both a critique and an alternative philosophy of practice they also engage in theory and argument.

So, in this chapter, I will examine some theories underpinning the concepts of autonomy and respect for persons. In doing so, I shall locate the principles and values of palliative care setting the ground for chapter 5 and a more practical approach to autonomy.

Theorizing the philosophy of palliative care

Perhaps it is naïve to think that there could be a distinct philosophy of palliative care given the evolutionary changes palliative care has undergone from the early hospice movement to the present context of palliative medicine. If you look to the writings of the early pioneers of the modern hospice movement then there does seem to emerge a consistent and coherent set of values (Saunders 1959). In the previous chapter, I summarized these values and aspirations from Saunders introduction to the *Oxford Textbook of Palliative Medicine* (1993). These values have been variously woven into a 'philosophy' — in the sense of an ideology that has been summarized by the WHO rubric into a distinct philosophy statement. Although it is not clear that the WHO statement is a good summary of the values and principles I listed. In addition, the WHO statement contains a number of serious ambiguities.

Some commentators have been critical of the implication that palliative care is a distinct area of practice from the rest of medicine. In their 1999 book, Randall and Downie made the point that:

> Palliative care is not an 'island' of philosophy and practice for a few privileged patients and staff. It is an integral part of effective health care. Its aims and scope should therefore fall within those of health care, and its philosophy must be compatible with that of a comprehensive health service.
>
> (Randall and Downie 1999: 16)

In their 2006 book, Randall and Downie offer a detailed critique of the WHO (2002) 'philosophy' of palliative care and the forms of practice this represents. They also offer a new alternative, a distillation of their arguments from the 1999 book, which amounts to a thoroughly medicalized view succinctly expressed. When reflecting on the need for a philosophy statement Randall and Downie conclude that it must:

> ... be consistent with the aims, values and assumptions of health care in general. Secondly these aims should be consistent with professional aims and the law. It is essential that a new philosophy should not influence health care practitioners to act contrary to their professional codes and the law. Thirdly, the aims and values of palliative care should not cause its practitioners to pursue goals which are unattainable or inequitable in terms of the resources of a publicly funded health care system.
>
> (Randall and Downie 2006: 220)

Although Randall and Downie direct their arguments to palliative care, it is clear that their criticisms and arguments apply to all areas of medicine. In summary, what they promote is a reaffirmation of a quite traditional medical ethical view. This is, of course, not necessarily a criticism of that view, but it raises the possibility of a conflict with the frequently espoused belief that palliative care offers a discrete alternative philosophy.

The essence of Randall and Downie's position is as follows: any medical speciality, even though this may rely upon multi-disciplinary teamwork, centres upon the responsibility of the doctor since they have ultimate legal responsibility for the patient's treatment. The doctor–patient relationship is one that is premised upon the legal concept of consent that requires the doctor to provide the degree of information the patient requires to be informed enough to give meaningful consent to treatment. The Doctor's duty of care requires that she give the patient her whole attention during clinical contact and, moreover, should aspire to communicate in a friendly, but not intimate manner. This duty of care extends to the patient only and requires the doctor to respect the patient's confidentiality, relying upon their consent to disclose their medical details to family members. The treatment offered to the patient must, in her judgement, be to the benefit of the patient. Although she should respect the views of the patient she is not obliged to treat the patient in such a way that conflicts with her own view of the patient's good or the law. This, of course, is a philosophy that can be encountered in any medico-legal textbook!

What is curious about Randal and Downie's 'new philosophy' is that, with the exception of the paragraph that defines palliative care, there is nothing that singles the philosophy out as unique and special to palliative care. In particular, there is nothing within the philosophy that conveys the essence of the 'quiet art' they themselves believe their philosophy conveys. What I say is also, of course, equally true of the WHO statement. Perhaps the detail is to be found in what they argue in the body of their book. This is also true of other writings on palliative care, and I have related in earlier chapters some of the ideals and values that have been consistently championed from the hospice movement onwards. One idea frequently discussed by Cicely Saunders in her writings and letters, is the idea that the dying person is on a journey with the potential for a therapeutic relationship between carer and patient, and offering the potential for all members of the team to be equally involved. The object of the journey is the possibility of peace and reconciliation with death. Although this form of good death had specifically a Christian context for Cicely Saunders, it became apparent that this was personal to her and not to all others. However, the challenge of helping all dying people to achieve their version of the good death has been an abiding value and one that has necessitated listening to patients, eliciting their preferences and attempting to respond with an appropriate package of care. Although the overtly religious connotation has gone, this value is discernible in the NHS end-of-life programme described in the previous chapter. To maintain the belief that a task of palliative care is to enable a person to achieve their own good death requires the capacity to adapt over time; to keep pace with social change and values. To take the belief seriously also requires an engagement with individual autonomy, which is not at a superficial level, but is linked with a deeper understanding of what it is to show respect for individuals. Randall and Downie quickly dismiss contemporary notions of autonomy as overemphasized contrivances of liberal values and consumer rights (2006: 9). I agree that the concept of autonomy has become bloated within contemporary medical ethics but there is a deeper analysis to be made. So-called 'consumer autonomy' has its roots in the established and pervasive political philosophy of liberalism. So in order to critique and perhaps dismiss consumer autonomy as irrelevant to the way respect for individuals ought to be shown, in palliative care, in health care and, more generally, requires some analysis.

The dominant discourse within contemporary western medical ethics is liberal secularism (Savulescu 1997; Beauchamp and Childress 2003). In a nutshell, this means that medical ethics is premised upon a system of negative rights, such as freedom from interference and freedom from harm albeit against a background of beneficent intent. This is the position I take as being implicit within both of Randall and Downie's books. The standard formulation of the set of values or principles that informs liberal medical ethics is the framework of Four Principles as described by Beauchamp and Childress (2003):

- Autonomy: principle of respect for autonomy.
- Non-maleficence: principle of avoiding harm to others.
- Beneficence: principle of doing good.
- Justice: principle of fairness and equality.

Although many critics, and Beauchamp and Childress in their own commentary, have warned against a too-formulaic use of this framework; the framework does appear to be ubiquitous as a formula for teaching health care ethics. Indeed, Randall and Downie make the point that they specifically wish to avoid using such a formula because health professionals never use such theories when faced with a practical moral problem (2006: 14). I agree, as this is an observation consistent with the pragmatic approach. People generally act and behave in certain ways out of habit. Novices entering a profession, like nursing or medicine, learn how to be a professional by learning the habits of the profession. However, it is only when one wishes to challenge or change such habits that a mechanism for stepping outside the habit is needed. Routine paternalism in medicine was just such a habit that needed challenging. Using concepts such as autonomy as theoretical tools encouraged critical reflection upon established practises. This is, of course, put too simplistically. However, my point is that, through critical reflection on practises, using theoretical concepts it is possible to introduce a mechanism by which to examine established habits and practises, and this is exactly the activity that Randall and Downie are engaged in. It may be the case that respect for autonomy has itself become an overused habit and, therefore, the concept has become blunted as a tool for reflection (Clauser and Gert 1999). I claimed earlier that theories do not drive moral practises, it is also the case that, from the perspective of moral practises that *do* seem to work, it is possible to challenge theories that do not sit well with those moral practises. Perhaps the time to be most alarmed is when practises and theory coincide too comfortably. On this point, there is, in fact, a great deal of similarity between Randall and Downie's philosophy and the Four Principles approach they eschew. Within their proposed new philosophy of palliative care their emphasis on consent and respect for patient's refusals sits within the principle of respect for autonomy. Their risk/benefits approach to the appropriateness of treatment sits within the principles of beneficence and non-maleficence, and their attention to fairness is entirely consistent with the principlist approach to justice.

Ethics and values

As discussed in chapter 1, a central task of ethics is to establish what sort of 'thing' has moral value and, as a branch of philosophy, this task also involves the questioning of prior assumptions. Hence, in Plato's many dialogues you will witness Socrates challenging his interlocutors to define and defend key moral concepts. Of course, moral discourse is not the sole preserve of philosophy and nor is it, within philosophy, merely the task of conceptual analysis. However, in contrast to philosophy, which tries to be explicit and critical, other discourses are often implicit, and describe, rather than critically evaluate, the values by which they are informed. This is true, to an extent, of commentators on palliative care, and I have described in chapter 3 how the early contributors to palliative care expressed a vocational calling to deal with the suffering of dying patients. That there is a duty to respond to human suffering is perhaps unremarkable given that human values are rooted in human experience and suffering is generally seen as something to be ameliorated. Explicit recognition of this duty has a long history, being present in both Hippocratic and Christian traditions. This observation applies also to health care ethics were the presumption is that it is humans, who have moral significance and are of primary concern. However, philosophical scrutiny of these ethical presumptions has raised challenging and important questions. The fact of human suffering goes unchallenged, but the ethical response to suffering has been articulated from a number of different ethical perspectives. A consistent vein of thought in Hippocratic medical ethics has been the duality of beneficence and non-maleficence, the first duty being to do no harm, then to do good if at all possible. Historically the arbiter of what constitutes harm and benefit was the doctor, who also determined what was to be done; this was the essence of paternalism. The paternalistic approach in medicine has long since been challenged and a number of forces have been at play in this challenge. The growing awareness of individual rights as political and legal concepts, the ubiquity in the west of consumerism and consumer rights, and the recognition of such rights in the form of a moral principle, respect for autonomy, have all challenged paternalism in its various forms. The emphasis on rights has set up a tension between medicine's traditional concern with welfare and doing good, and the now pervasive demand to respect individual autonomy. In western medicine, the trend has been to resolve this tension in favour of respect for autonomy with the implication that respecting a person's autonomy has greater moral weight than advancing their welfare. For those who place a high premium on autonomy, welfare considerations have no or only minor significance in determining what is good for a person, hence, Harris's claim:

> So autonomy, as the ability and the freedom to make the choices that shape our lives, is quite crucial in giving to each life its own special and peculiar value ... So that where concern for welfare and respect for wishes are incompatible one with another, concern for welfare must give way to respect for autonomy.
>
> (Harris 1995: 11)

For Harris, the welfare of a person, even their very life are legitimate trade-offs in order that a person's autonomy be respected. In a similar vein, Dworkin argues that the value of autonomy is independent of considerations of an agent's welfare since:

> ... autonomy encourages and protects the capacity competent people have to direct their own lives at least generally in accordance with a scheme of value each has recognised and chosen for himself or herself.
>
> (Dworkin 1986: 9)

On the basis of these kinds of consideration, it is argued by many that respect for autonomy is therefore crucial to the moral respect for persons. Hence, autonomy ought to be given high regard in the context of healthcare, where many of the decisions made will influence the length and quality of a person's life.

As discussed in chapter 1, alongside the growing emphasis on individual rights and autonomy, there has also been a challenge to the premise that human individuals in virtue of being *human* have intrinsic moral worth (Harris 1983; Singer 1995). The philosophical debate has centred upon the criteria for moral worth and whether this is an essence, being human, or whether it is the possession of particular *properties*, which individual human beings may or may not have. Which of these criteria are accepted has implications for the extent of moral duties with quite particular implications for palliative care. In secular liberal ethics, there has been a move towards the view that merely being human is not sufficient to establish the moral status of a thing. I believe this is a mistaken view. The contrasting belief, that human value is divinely ordained, one of the mainstays of traditional medical ethics, is also problematic in a world in which the duties and responsibilities of the state are expected to be secular in nature.

The liberal view on human moral status is one approach to arguing for the kind of political organization of contemporary society. Although the liberal view is not universally accepted, it is a view that drives many of the contemporary moral debates. These debates are played out in response to the ever-new challenges that medical research and new technology pose for contemporary living. The scientific knowledge and medical know-how that resulted in the birth of Louise Brown, the first 'test-tube' baby contributed directly to the development of embryo research and the possibility of human cloning. In doing so, the developments created as much ethical controversy at the beginning of life as the invention of the artificial respirator did at the end of life. Medical knowledge and technology has disturbed the foundations of the twin pillars, which mark the boundaries of human mortality, birth and death. Although for those who are inclined to accept the primacy of autonomy, the debate has allegedly clarified the boundaries, rather than confused them.

The liberal view of autonomy I have outlined regards both the living embryo and the living, but permanently comatose patient as having the status of living human tissues, rather than morally valuable individuals (Harris 1983; Parfit 1991; Singer 1994). Parfit states:

> ... a person can gradually cease to exist some time before his heart stops beating. This will be so if the distinctive features of a person's mental life gradually disappear. This often happens. We can plausibly claim that, if the person has ceased to exist, we have no moral reason to help his heart to go on beating, or to refrain from preventing this.
>
> This claim distinguishes the person from the human being. If we know that a human being is in a coma that is incurable — that this human being will never regain consciousness — we shall believe that the person shall cease to exist. Since there is a living human body, the human being exists. But, at this end of lives, we should claim that only the killing of persons is wrong.
>
> (Parfit 1991: 323)

This is the kind of argument that underpins the *persons* approach to moral significance that I discussed in chapter 1. The implication of accepting this view is that a number of established moral conventions are radically challenged, for example, the idea that, in medicine, there is a duty of care to promote the best interests of the patient no matter what capacity they possess. The logical force of the autonomy argument is often regarded as morally counter-intuitive because most people do not believe themselves relieved of moral responsibility for the permanently unconscious or incapacitated patient merely because they lack certain capacities.

Although these are not necessarily the issues that spring to the fore as the central ethical challenges in palliative care, how a principle of respect for autonomy ought to be interpreted is. One can readily observe the many ways in which respect for autonomy is manifest in palliative care through certain routine practises. The aspiration to care for a patient with open disclosure and honest communication, the facilitation of patients in planning a realistic future and by offering choice so far as services can support those choices.

In other areas, there are more palpable tensions, for example, when patient and family disagree about what is best, when individual choices about what ought to happen to their dying or no longer competent self cannot be supported, and where palliative options contradict an individual's willingness to risk high stakes in treatment for a small chance of benefit. Recent legal cases in the UK and other jurisdictions have shown that patients and families are unwilling to allow medicine to arbitrate over what is and is not appropriate for individuals (Boyd 2002; Gostin 2005). This represents one of the real challenges for palliative care. It is a challenge, which according to Randall and Downie, the speciality has failed to meet, with practitioners routinely caving in to patient's 'consumer rights' (2006: 10).

Respect for autonomy is echoed in law by the recognition of the right to self-determination and it is therefore not surprising that such a principle should have gained a prominent place within contemporary health care ethics. Respect for autonomy gains something approaching legal force because it is acknowledged as underpinning several of the important foundations to ethical professional practice such as consent and confidentiality.

Liberalism, autonomy and the good life

In chapter 2, I introduced some discussion of theories of the good life or axiology, I shall now turn to consider a number of theoretical approaches beginning with the liberal approach. Liberal thinkers particularly hold the right to self-determination in high regard (Kymlicka 1990). Although liberals and non-liberals alike may acknowledge that we are all engaged in the process of pursuing the best sort of life for ourselves, the liberal view, as philosophers such as Mill and Rawls have argued, is that no one is in a better position than the person him or herself to determine what is good for them (Kymlicka 1990). The implication of this position is that the best form of political and social order is one that supports maximum individual autonomy, since it is only by maximizing personal liberty that individuals are free to pursue and revise their own view about what is valuable in life. This is a position that has become highly pervasive in governments, institutions and within practises including health care. It is a viewpoint that has important implications for the palliative care community, and the implicit and explicit values it endorses.

While there is, of course, no single uncontested account of autonomy the liberal approach is consistent and I shall now trace its origins (Holm 1995; Clauser and Gert 1999; Woods 2005).

Like most complex concepts the meaning of autonomy is evolving. Its ancient origin lies in Greek political theory, where autonomy literally meant self-governing or self-legislation, but the modern accounts of autonomy have moved on from this context. Human history, since that time, has witnessed a repeated endeavour to define what it is to be a morally significant entity. An aspect of the contemporary meaning of autonomy is therefore interwoven with a modern understanding of the 'self' and individuality that, to an extent, have become moral cornerstones in contemporary *western* thinking. Although I emphasize 'western' it is also true that the belief in the importance of individual autonomy is not embraced by everyone in the west, since the west consists of diverse cultures. However, to an extent, this diversity is compatible with the liberal approach, since liberals support the political view that the best societies are those that allow for the greatest diversity. A commitment to autonomy is therefore the basis of such a political structure.

Autonomy, understood as self-rule, is tied to the modern concept of 'self', a complex construct, closely tied to concepts of liberty and freedom, identity and individualism. Immanuel Kant (1786), probably the first modern thinker to address autonomy, saw the freedom to act autonomously as a necessary condition for moral action. The Kantian view, as Farsides puts it, is that: 'the most valuable form of autonomy entails voluntarily choosing to do that which is right' (Farsides 1998: 148). The Kantian view of autonomy is also endorsed by Randall and Downie (2006), but to insist that autonomy should only be understood from a Kantian perspective ignores the social and philosophical changes, which now contribute to its contemporary meaning and usage.

This is not to dismiss the Kantian version of autonomy as irrelevant. However, to do justice to the detail of Kant's approach requires an enquiry that is beyond the purposes of this book. However, the broad brush of the Kantian account of the autonomous self does provide an understanding of the moral *equivalence* of individuals. Autonomous individuals are worthy of equal respect and, therefore, a community of autonomous individuals must comply with a principle of mutual respect. In summary, the two key aspects of Kantian autonomy is that to be autonomous requires a capacity to deliberate on the good and that autonomous individuals are of equal moral worth. Both aspects of the Kantian approach to autonomy became a key feature of the theory of autonomy, which liberal thinkers then took further.

For Liberals like John Stuart Mill (1859), each *individual*, and by this is meant something like each competent adult, is sovereign to himself and ought therefore to be treated as free to decide for himself. This liberal conception of freedom is essentially a *negative* one, thus, the freedom from interference becomes central to liberal autonomy, except where one person's actions pose a threat to the safety and security of others. The negative version of autonomy, emphasizing freedom *from* interference does not require a substantive account of what it is right to do. The implication of this version of autonomy is that individual choices and the ends they aim at are of equal value, so long as the means used to pursue those ends allows an equal degree of freedom for others to pursue their own choices and ends. Thus, we can distinguish between two senses of autonomy, the Kantian sense in which autonomous action is freely choosing to do the right thing and the liberal account in which *respect* for autonomy entails non-interference in the choices of others. It is therefore possible to see, in this change in the meaning of autonomy, the seeds of the version of autonomy, 'consumer autonomy' rightly condemned by Randall and Downie.

Although the principle of non-interference has become widely recognized in law and medicine it is not entirely on the basis that all choices and goals are of equal value. There is a sense that there is some constraint on what can be advocated as a 'good' way of living. However, the ability to say in any constructive way what this might mean is becoming increasingly difficult in a world of diverse values. This negative formulation of autonomy poses a specific challenge for medicine, since the call to respect individual choice stands in conflict with the aspiration of medicine to actually do good for individual patients and for populations in the face of the range of lifestyle choices that are often patently bad for people. Medicine or at least, health care can be regarded in one of two ways. One is to view health care as the means of pursuing a substantive common good 'health' which can be legitimately pursued even at the expense of other goods and values including, perhaps, the value of individual autonomy. The second is to see health care as a means of enabling social justice by removing or preventing one of the barriers to individual freedom, ill-health, and, hence, enabling individuals to pursue their own life. The liberalization of health care ethics has meant a shift from the paternalism of the former to the autonomy focus of the latter.

The question here is whether palliative care has undergone a similar transition towards liberal values with regard to what constitutes a good death? The idea that some substance can be given to the 'good death' has and indeed continues to have an influence on the values of palliative care. Although the notion that the good death is one that is pain free, peaceful, reconciled with family and accepting of death is now recognized as overly idealized, there is a sense in which the ideal is preserved as an inspiration to practice (Callahan 1993; McNamara *et al.* 1994; Copp 1998). The ideal may be too optimistic in terms of what medicine can achieve, has the potential to be overly prescriptive to individuals and demand too much of palliative care services (Randall and Downie 2006). Nevertheless, the ideal remains evident in, for example, Saunders introduction to the *Oxford Textbook of Palliative Medicine* (2005).

There have been many attempts through empirical research to be realistic with regard to what the dying process is like. Awareness of the reality of dying has led to the recognition that if palliative care sees its success only in terms of the ideal, a peaceful reconciled death, then it is set up to fail in what it does. This has resulted in a growing tendency to reflect upon and deconstruct the idealized good death. There is now a growing recognition that the good death cannot be given a meaningful substantive definition and, hence, negative constructions of the good death have come to the fore. The notion of articulating the aim of palliative care in terms of achieving the 'least worst' or 'good enough' death has become increasingly common (McNamara 1998; Randall and Downie 1999). However, if the good death can no longer be constructed in terms of a set of positive ideals then there is a challenge for the construction of palliative care, is it merely there to facilitate the patient's choice or to advocate a way of dying? To accept the former, is to accept a liberal value set.

I believe that this is part of the dilemma for contemporary palliative care. However, I also believe that a case can be made for a distinct palliative care axiology, which I have begun to characterize and now develop in more detail in the second part of this chapter.

In drawing a parallel between liberal accounts of autonomy, and the goals and values of medicine and palliative care, I have drawn attention to two approaches to understanding the 'good' life. The Kantian approach emphasizes the importance of the autonomous 'deliberating' individual freely doing what ought to be done. The broadly liberal approach I have described offers a negative account of the good life in terms of the constraints with which we are required to comply in order to allow an equal degree of freedom for others to live by their own choices. If these two accounts seem similar, then that is because of an ambiguity in the meaning of 'good' in the context of the 'good life'. The difference can be understood if one considers two kinds of question, the first concerns the kind of life we *wish* to live, the second concerns the kind of life we *ought* to live. In the Kantian case, the 'good life' has as its focus a concern with the life we ought to live, in the sense of what ought we to do to live a morally good life. Here, the principal focus is on the individual who must willingly decide to do what is right in order to live the morally good life.

The liberal approach addresses the question of the 'good life' by considering the kind of life the individual wishes to live in terms of the goodness or qualities of a life that make life enjoyable and worthwhile. From the liberal point of view there are no universal truths with respect to the good life, no 'givens' in terms of religious revelation about how to live and, therefore, people should be free to pursue their own conception of the good life. The moral implication for liberals is to consider the set of social or political arrangements that allow individuals an equal degree of freedom to pursue their own conception of the good life, rather than having a conception imposed upon them. It is through these arrangements that ethical constraints are identified, and pre-eminent for liberals is respect for individual autonomy.

I shall now develop this discussion further by the use of a number of practical examples some of which are based upon publicly discussed cases.

In 2002, a woman known as Ms B was admitted to a UK hospital following a haemorrhage into her cervical spine. The injury left her permanently paralysed below the neck and unable to breathe independently. After several months in this condition she eventually requested that the ventilator be removed. Ms B's medical carers were unwilling to comply and at first declared her to lack the capacity to make such a decision. In other words, they judged her to lack the autonomous capacity to make such a judgement. Ms B had not left the confines of the intensive care unit in which she was situated and she refused to consider rehabilitation because, whatever support was available to her, nothing could be done to alleviate her absolute dependence on a ventilator and physical care. This was not in her view a life worth living even though some of her carers and individuals in similar circumstances claimed that there was a possibility of living a worthwhile life. The dispute went to Court, which found in Ms B's favour (Boyd 2002; Stauch 2002). The judgement made in this case suggested that no person should be compelled to comply with a health care regime, even though this was believed to be in their best interests. This case involved a patient's refusal of life-sustaining treatment. This, and similar cases, are often used as exemplars of how autonomy or the right to self-determination is instantiated in Law. Such cases are also used to dismiss parallel moral claims in which a person demands a service or resource for themselves where they believe such a service or resource *is* in their interests, based upon their own deeply held convictions. The standard legal and perhaps also moral approach is to argue that there is a profound difference between an individual refusing life-sustaining treatment and a person requesting a positive intervention to end their life. In giving evidence to the House of Lords committee on the *Assisted Dying for the Terminally Ill Bill,* John Finnis described this distinction as the 'bright line' (House of Lords 2005b II:

553). Although Finnis also believes that the case of Ms B transgressed this line, others strive to maintain that there are profound differences between removing a ventilator and giving a lethal injection; an analysis that makes the line less bright than fragile.

I have used this example because it serves to illustrate three different ways of making the case for how constraints may be justifiably applied to autonomous wishes. The first is demonstrated by the Finnis approach, who as a Catholic and academic lawyer is well known to defend the doctrine of sanctity of life. On this view, autonomous wishes to bring about death ought to be refused. This is the position I believe is closest to the hospice opposition to euthanasia and assisted dying. The second position is that which respects autonomous refusals of life-sustaining treatment, accepting the consequences of such decisions, but believing that this is an appropriate measure of respect for a person. This is the position I believe is most consistent with contemporary palliative care, and is certainly the view endorsed by Randall and Downie (2006). The third position is the one advocated by Dworkin (1993), Harris (1995) and others that, in this instance, we ought to respect a person's autonomous wish and assist their death; a position that is still generally opposed.

I believe that there are a number of forces at play, which account for the transition from the early hospice position on euthanasia and assisted dying to the current position. One is the loosening of the attachment to a religiously grounded sanctity of life position and another is the acceptance of a more liberal approach to respect for persons. I suggest that what has prevented a complete acceptance of liberal autonomy and its implications for end of life decisions is that the palliative care community has managed to maintain an overarching axiology, which is resistant to liberalism. I shall now set out my case for this claim.

Palliative care axiology

The analysis I have so far offered of liberal accounts of autonomy suggests that liberalism places great emphasis upon the individual as an authority on his or her own good. Critics argue that this plays down the significance of the person as situated in a social and relational context (Mulhall and Swift 1997). This alternative view to liberalism, although made up of quite diverse thinkers, is known collectively as 'communitarianism' (Kymlicka 1990) Communitarianism can be defined in terms of the criticisms it makes of the liberal position and in terms of a number of positive alternative claims. Both aspects are relevant as possible frameworks for understanding palliative care values.

Liberals value autonomy because liberals are sceptical with regard to there being any single account of what constitutes a good life for a person to lead (Kymlicka 1990). This stands in contrast to the communitarian positions, which like religious and other ancient philosophical beliefs, takes the view that the good life for human beings can be captured in terms of an over-arching framework of values that gives both meaning and purpose to life.

In chapter 2, I introduced the concept of axiology as the branch of philosophy, which deals with theories of the good life. The 'good life' means the form of life that will enable a person to flourish or live well. In contemporary philosophical analysis this has come to be considered as a question about self-interest, what makes a life go well for *me*? (Parfit 1991). There are, of course, an abundance of religious and political theories that purport to provide the definitive account, and many do so in terms of the end or purpose of human life; these are termed teleological accounts. The Ancient Greek philosopher Aristotle offered rationality or reason, as the *telos* or goal, as the good life for man (Kenny 1992). Like the Aristotelian version, axiological theories have often attempted to give a reductionist account of the good life in terms of a single criterion. I have argued that for liberals autonomy has something of this role because there is no single authoritative view about the good life for humans other than that determined by the individual. Autonomy or freedom to choose for oneself is therefore crucial to this enterprise. It is also why this view requires a sufficient account of how and in what terms individuals can be said to have such an authoritative view of their own lives. In chapter 2, I also explored different approaches to subjective axiology. Subjective approaches attempt to account for the goodness of a life either in terms of the quality of a person's experiences, or in terms of the satisfaction a person feels when their life is going well according to their wishes and preferences. These are powerful accounts because they appeal to what is familiar to each of us, namely the seeming authoritative ability to evaluate one's own experiences. However, there are many problems with this approach, but two are relevant to our interests here. First, although such theories may identify plausible and necessary components of a good life, they are far from sufficient to guarantee a good life (Sandman 2005). That is, one may be living a pleasing or satisfying life yet still regard that life, when regarded from another perspective, as falling below a standard. The second challenges the idea that the good life consists of a life devoted to the pursuit of pleasurable experiences or the satisfaction of desires *per se*. This is because that, on reflection, these seem quite unconvincing accounts of the good life.

Pleasurable experiences are, tautologically, *good*, but only if we are satisfied that pleasure and goodness are synonymous. Pleasurable experiences may be part of, indeed essential to a good life, but a life that consists of nothing but the pursuit of pleasurable experiences seems to be lacking as a complete account of the good life. Part of the problem is that there needs to be a very rich account of what 'pleasure' means for such accounts to be compatible with our common sense conception of a good life. In chapter 2, I also explored the possibility of using drugs to induce pleasant mental states as a means to achieving a good dying. I rejected this possibility because pleasure, construed as a pleasing sensation, is very one-dimensional, and might be regarded as something fleeting and superficial, trivial even. In life, we do distinguish between different kinds of pleasure, or at least between the sensations enjoyed, and the context and meaning with which the pleasure is associated. Indeed, the 'pleasures' that seem to be most valued can hardly be described as pleasures at all. The 'pleasure' of achieving an athletic or sporting goal like competing in the Olympic Games requires a great deal of personal sacrifice, pain even. This kind of achievement requires planning and foresight. It also requires the ability to acknowledge that individual successes and failures are part of a coherent whole, the sum of which is greater than the individual parts. This example goes some way to modelling an account of a candidate good life, since it reflects complexity, a diversity of ends, with a role for purpose and value which makes talk of 'pleasure' as the *raison d'être* seem overly simplistic.

Similarly, there are limitations on the extent to which the goodness of one's life is truly reflected in the level of satisfaction one experiences. The claim that the goodness of a life is judged by the feeling of satisfaction that we enjoy when our preferences and wishes are fulfilled may be challenged on two fronts, first with regard to the importance of the *feeling* of satisfaction and, second, with regard to the preferences themselves. For example, it is not difficult to imagine feeling satisfied that one's desire has been fulfilled yet being mistaken that the conditions of satisfaction have been met. Take, for example, the sort of scene a medical television soap opera might depict: a character in his death throes is desperately hanging on for a visit from his son for what he hopes will be a final reconciliation. The son does not arrive, but the patient mistakes a kindly doctor for his son, and the doctor plays the part and listens to the patient's dying apology and attempt at reconciliation, after which he dies 'satisfied,' believing that his reconciliation is real. This scene provokes a number of thoughts; for example, does it matter that the doctor merely played the part? Surely the dying man made his gesture and died satisfied? The problem is this, if we take seriously the claim that the good life is one in which we feel satisfied that our desires have been fulfilled then, on this account, there can be no reason to choose between two possible worlds; one in which we merely believe our desires satisfied and one in which they really are satisfied. However, this equivalence does not seem to hold, since we do believe that authenticity and truth matter, and are anxious that we do not lead our lives on the basis of false beliefs and so the world in which our desires really have been met seems objectively better (Raz 1986). What this at least shows is that it is not merely in virtue of feeling satisfied that our desires are met that our life goes best. One may argue that the implications for our dying man are that it is better, both for him and the doctor that he is aware of the reality of his situation, even though this may frustrate his desire.

There are also problems, however, with the claim that the good life consists in having one's desires or preferences actually satisfied. With regard to preferences, it seems reasonable to accept a person's choices and desires as an authentic account of their preferences. However, it is odd to claim that what is good for a person, what gives them the best sort of life, does so simply because they *choose* it and are then satisfied when their choice is fulfilled. It is clear that the goodness of the life of a person can be judged poor, even if many of his or her wishes and preferences are satisfied, because their set of preferences are meagre. It is not the mere number of desire/satisfaction pairings that make a life go better, as Parfit (1991) has shown it is possible to increases the number of desires we have that are satisfied in our daily life, but if these desires are trifling then no matter how many of these desires are satisfied they do not add to the quality of a person's life in a significant way. However, if this is obvious in trivial cases, it is much less so in more complex cases, and the issue of who is to judge and on what grounds has been of long-term concern to liberal thinkers.

Dworkin (1993) draws attention to the possibility of judging the goodness of a life independently of its 'felt' qualities. Dworkin describes this as a distinction between an individual's 'experiential interests' and their overarching or abiding interests, which give shape and meaning to a life. This distinction suggests the possibility of an objective theory of axiology, but how are these issues played out in the palliative care context?

Thinking in this philosophical way about the nature of the good life is rarely done so explicitly within the palliative care literature. However, the palliative care literature does discuss theories, as well as describe particular case histories aimed to make the point that a person's own judgement of the quality of their life can be improved upon, for example, by patients who achieve peace, reconciliation and acceptance when they were initially resistant to the idea of palliative care (Kubler-Ross 1969; Kearney 1992; Billings 1998). Of course, the aim of palliative care is not to argue at a theoretical level only, but to show that palliative care is effective practically. However, how this is shown is deeply problematic. Randall and Downie (2006) have argued that a consequence of an uncritical adoption of Hippocratic medicine has resulted in an obsession with quantification, assessment and gathering of pseudo-scientific evidence. The problem with this indiscriminate approach is that it does not distinguish between different kinds of evidence. Evidence of a robust scientific kind is needed to show that a drug is efficacious or that one drug is better than another. This sort of evidence may be used to persuade a patient that taking an opiate drug will be better for their pain, and will not harm them. However, what sort of *evidence* might be used to convince a person in the advanced stages of a terminal illness, refusing admission to a hospice because of their own preconvictions about hospices? Palliative care practitioners are convinced that, if this person can be persuaded to try palliative care, then they will see for themselves that their life will be or at least has the opportunity to be better. Changing a person's convictions and attempting to win their trust is not a case of presenting a portfolio of evidence. Making the case for palliative care is to present a possibility, an opportunity for the person to see that there might be a better way of dying. However, to do this with sincerity the opportunity cannot come with promises because palliative care cannot be offered with a promise that things will be better. Cicely Saunders couched this potential cautiously as '[t]he often surprising potential for personal and family growth' (2005: xix). This potential within palliative care is, however, presented as a plausible case in which it is possible to judge the goodness of a life objectively; that palliative care offers an objectively better way of dying than the alternatives, including euthanasia. It might therefore be argued that it is reasonable to attempt to persuade the reluctant patient to try palliative care in order to see for themselves that things might be better. This is not, of course, an argument justifying the *imposition* of palliative care upon patients, although it gives a clue as to how a principle of respect for autonomy might be understood in the context of palliative care. The most difficult case is where the patient believes that they have a superior alternative in that they wish their life to end sooner, rather than later. I shall return to such cases in subsequent chapters.

The idea that palliative care offers a genuine alternative together with an acknowledgement of the limitations of that offer is something that has clearly influenced Randall and Downie's (2006) new philosophy of palliative care. Palliative care can promise a high standard of professional clinical care from specialists with expertize in symptom management. It cannot promise, in Randall and Downie's view, the 'softer' goods of spiritual and psycho-social care, and treatment of the whole family, it cannot promise the peaceful and reconciled death. This, of course, is a radically altered presentation of palliative care and put in these terms there is little to distinguish it from other medical specialities.

The possibility of an objective axiology requires some unpacking. One sense of 'objective' is to claim that there are certain necessary components of a good life independent of the experiences of the individual. As discussed in chapter 2, these are often expressed, particularly by liberal thinkers such as Rawls (1971), in a 'thin' way as general abstract qualities, health, nourishment, liberty and so on. A second sense of 'objective' is concerned with the nature of judgement and the possibility of making a reasoned case that one thing is, all things considered, *better* than another.

This approach does not give immediate priority to the judgements of the person whose life it is, but allows the possibility that their view might be moved on as a consequence of being presented with a different conception of what is good. This is how I conceive that the palliative care alternative can be most meaningfully presented.

Between different people there are differences of opinion about the relative value and importance of different lifestyles that cannot be resolved by appeal to objective qualities in the first sense of objective. People do have different views and beliefs, different ideas about what constitutes a good life in their own case. It is also possible to accept that such beliefs and the plans they give rise to could be revised for the better. The liberal view is that because there is no absolute authority with regard to what is good, then priority ought to be given to the individual to make the judgement about their own good life. As Jeremy Waldron suggests it is an axiom of liberalism: '... that there is something like *pursuing a conception of the good life* that all people, even those with the most diverse commitments, can be said to be engaged in' (Waldron 1987: 145).

The liberal view does not amount to a denial of objective goods in the first sense, but rather that any objective conception of the good must not impose a particular kind of life upon individuals (Rawls 1971). The political implication of this view is that the state, in its widest sense, should not impose or endorse a particular conception of the good.

The application of axiological theory is always in a particular political context and must inevitably engage therefore with ethics. Since it is not enough to consider in what way a life may be judged as a good life without considering the sort of life it is permissible to pursue. The question is whether this is achieved by condemning certain kinds of lifestyle and advocating others or by admitting the widest possible range of ways of living that can be mutually sustained. Generally, the liberal view regards a person's own good as insufficient grounds for interference in that person's life, but many believe some ways of living ought to be condemned and a person's right to pursue such a life restricted. However, liberals generally only favour proscription where one person's lifestyle has implications for *others* and not the interests of the individual concerned.

The liberal position has had a dominant place in this exploration of axiology because of the importance ascribed to autonomy in contemporary ethics relies on such an axiology as a rationale. Although I have argued that palliative care draws on an axiology rooted in communitarianism. This approach recognizes autonomy, but within a more general ethic of respect for persons. Communitarianism can be construed both as a critique of liberalism and as a positive alternative. These critics of liberalism are disturbed by the negative vision of humanity that it implies (Mulhall and Swift 1997). It is argued that, at its extreme, liberalism presents a very negative view of society as a colony of individuals engaged in competitive negotiations with other equally independent individuals, attempting to agree the set of compromises that will secure the best sort of life for themselves. In this version of society the only shared ideal is merely the set of compromises.

Communitarian criticisms of liberalism focus mainly upon how liberals construe the nature of the individual and how individuals come to a judgement about the nature of the good life. Both aspects can be contrasted to how communitarians construe the role of the self in the context of society. Liberals have an 'unencumbered' view of the self, a view that persists from Kant through Mill to Rawls (Kymlicka 1990). Kant advocated the view that the self was distinct from and prior to its social role, and hence the self could stand back and apply reason in the process of determining the right thing to do. Communitarians regard this as a false view of the self because it fails to consider the social context of practises and values from which it is not always possible to step back. As Mulhall and Swift comment, these criticisms do:

> ... not entail that individual autonomy should be altogether scrapped or entirely downgraded as a human good. It is rather designed to question the absoluteness of the priority and the universality of the scope that liberals are prone to assign to that good; it serves to suggest that both the priority and the scope should be modified or restricted.
>
> (Mulhall & Swift 1997: 163)

Communitarians object to the liberal view of the self as too abstract, artificially removed, and isolated from the community from which it takes its identity and purpose. The charge is that liberal thought has been too influenced by a Kantian view of the self, which emphasizes the self's power of rational deliberation and its isolation from any context in its consideration of what is good. These features are clearly recognizable in John Rawls's thought experiment, where he imagines a group of citizens reflecting upon the principles of justice behind a 'veil of ignorance', where they are 'unencumbered' by knowledge of their actual role, talents and handicaps (Rawls 1971). Rawls summarizes his view as the claim that 'the self is prior to the ends which are affirmed by it' (1971: 560). The liberal position is that the self both defines and constrains those ends, whereas the communitarians maintain that it is what is already known, what is shared, which helps both to define and place limits on how the good is defined (MacIntyre 1981). In comparison to the 'neutral' view of the good assumed by liberals, communitarians are said to be 'perfectionist' to the extent that certain ways of life are said to constitute the good ('perfection') and should be promoted by the state and its various institutions.

The task of this chapter has been to explore the concept of autonomy, the relevance of the principle of respect for autonomy in ethics and in the context of palliative care particularly. Autonomy is closely tied to a concept of the self, of the individual, and I have set out how a liberal interpretation of this suggests a particular approach to showing respect for persons. In brief, the liberal position accepts that it is the individual alone who defines their own good and, therefore, to respect the person, one must respect the decisions they make for themselves. In essence, the liberal view is that people matter because they are capable of valuing. This contrasts with the position taken within palliative care where respect for persons requires more than valuing the person's capacity for autonomy. On this view, people matter because they are *valuable,* a point that is reiterated in many of the affirmations of the palliative care community, but is most succinctly summed up in Saunders: 'You matter because you are you, and you matter until the last moment of your life' (2003: 46).

This, I suggest, places palliative care ethics in line with a communitarian approach. The dying person whose capacity for autonomy gradually diminishes, remains the focus of care, empathy and help. This sort of value is an example of something deeply ingrained and one that has become a shared pursuit of that community. To value the person in this way is not something that has been arrived at through a process of reason, it is rather a starting point — an axiom of the approach.

The palliative care approach to the individual is itself embedded within a community of value, which has attempted to 'show' the good life by attending to the good death. This began with a Christian axiology, but is now expressed in secular communitarian terms. The question is whether, without the theological anchor, an ethical stance that is distinctive from liberal ethics can be sustained?

In chapter 3, I traced the history of the modern palliative care movement in which Christian Hospices established a template for the first modern hospice, St Christophers in 1967. In her early writing about the values upon which hospices were premised, Cicely Saunders continually wrote about the importance of 'place' and 'community' (Clark 1998). Saunders envisioned the hospice as a community of fellow travellers on a Christian journey or pilgrimage, where there was a sense of shared values and a common purpose. Saunders's writing also included reflections upon the nature and meaning of suffering, the mystery as to why a loving God would allow suffering, as well as the role of prayer. In her early writing there is a very explicit sense of a Christian axiology, but alongside this is the development of a set of values that come to be affirmed independently of Christian beliefs, values that appear distinctly communitarian in nature. These values include an early rejection of euthanasia, condemned not merely on the moral ground of the sanctity of life, but by showing, through case histories, that there is a 'better' alternative in ending one's life naturally, with opportunities for growth up to the last moment (Saunders 1959, 1976). It is clear that Saunders regards palliative care as not merely an alternative to, but a weapon against euthanasia, the rejection of which also provides an opportunity to affirm the value of individuals: 'Anything which says to the very ill or the very old that there is no longer anything that matters in their life would be a deep impoverishment to the whole of society' (1972: 20).

Other values include the emphasis of the context of the dying individual, embedded as they are in relationships with their family, carers and wider society. It goes without saying that effective and consistent symptom control were considered a prerequisite, but as instrumental to preventing despair and allowing the person the space to live until they died. In addition, honesty, open communication, spiritual and psychological care are all seen as essential values. These values and the vision of the good they endorse are summarized by Saunders in many places including the following from 1996, which seems to capture the positive account of the 'good':

> The advances in pharmacology are not the whole story... The search for meaning, for something in which to trust, may be expressed in many ways, direct and indirect, in metaphor or in silence, in gesture or in symbol or, perhaps most of all, in art and the unexpected potential for creativity at the end of life. Those who work in palliative care may have to realise that they too are being challenged to face this dimension for themselves. Many, both helper and patient, live in a secularized society and have no religious language. Some, will of course be in touch with their religious roots and find a familiar practice, liturgy or sacrament, to help their need. Others, however, will not. For them the insensitive suggestion by well meaning practitioners will be unwelcome. However if we can come not only in our professional capacity but in our common, vulnerable humanity there may be no need of words on our part, only of concerned listening. For those who do not wish to share their deepest needs, the way care is given can reach the most hidden places. Feelings of fear and guilt may seem inconsolable, but many of us have sensed that an inner journey has taken place and that a person nearing the end of life has found peace. Important relationships may be developed or reconciled at this time and a new sense of self worth develop.
>
> (Saunders 1996: 1601)

The emphasis which Saunders gives to 'place' not as a hospice building, but upon the palliative care community as a place or a community of shared values provides another parallel to communitarianism. Charles Taylor (1985), a communitarian philosopher, calls the priority given to social values in communitarianism the 'social thesis' and regards this as the antithesis of the liberal commitment to a state that is neutral as to the form of good it endorses. The communitarian position argues that it is only in a particular kind of society and social environment that the exercise of autonomy can be properly understood. As Kymlicka comments, Taylor's view is that: 'some limits on self-determination are required to preserve the social conditions which enable self-determination' (1990: 216). Taylor's view is perfectionist to the extent that the capacity to choose a conception of the good life can only be exercised within a community that advances a politics of the common good. As problematic as this view may be in general terms, it does seem to capture some of the intuitions about the good of palliative care, that advances positive values such that each person is valuable until they die, that there is value in dealing openly and honestly with challenging circumstances, that there is value in human relationships and potential for growth until death. There are also negative corollaries, such that individual autonomy is to be constrained in order that these other goods may be realized. These include the right to refuse treatment, but not demand specific treatments or other interventions including euthanasia, assisted suicide and deep sedation.

In a short paper written for the Hastings Centre Report (Saunders 1995) Cicely Saunders responds to the theme of conflicts of conscience in palliative care. The purpose of her paper is to reflect upon why, despite ongoing debate, the issues of euthanasia and physician-assisted suicide do not provoke the conflicts of conscience in Britain that they do elsewhere. The argument Saunders briefly develops is interesting in itself, but what is more interesting are the comments she makes about the nature of palliative care ethics and values. In a few short paragraphs, Saunders articulates a position in the language of contemporary bioethics that strongly reflects some of the most important communitarian values. In relation to autonomy, Saunders contrasts the liberal notion with a care approach when she says:

> The ethical principles of care have to balance patient autonomy or control with the justice owed to society as a whole. Our choices do not take place in a purely individual setting ...
>
> (Saunders 1995: 44)

My reading of this statement is that Saunders does not endorse the idea of the liberal 'unencumbered self', but notes the social context and the limits which that implies for individual autonomy. She goes on to say:

> But much remains still to do, guided by the principle that life is of value until its 'natural' end, with space for mending relationships and honouring important values, by competent ever-improving care ... As we have been vigorous in seeking ever better ways to help patients at the end of life, so I believe we can and should constantly reiterate that this is the way to respect patients' and families' true needs. Their autonomy must be seen in the context of society as a whole ...
>
> (Saunders 1995: 44)

Conclusion

I turn now to consider the place of palliative care within the spectrum between liberal and communitarian accounts of autonomy. One view of palliative care is to see no significant difference between palliative care and any other health discipline. On this narrow view, palliative care is just palliative *medicine* and, as such, accepts autonomy as part of the secular liberal spectrum that is arguably the foundation of contemporary medical ethics. This is, of course, a controversial account and one that continues to be debated within the field. It is perhaps nearer the truth to claim that, while it may not be entirely accurate to say that *palliative care* is synonymous with *palliative medicine* this state of affairs is becoming increasingly nearer the truth as palliative care evolves as a health speciality.

An alternative view sees the history of palliative care as standing outside that of health care and drawing explicitly upon a moral foundation of 'theological' axiology, rather than a secular liberal one. On this view, palliative care can be seen as having a transcendental axiology of its own, a vision of the good life that includes a particular view of the good death. Evidence for this can be seen in the religious and specifically Christian foundation of modern hospices that formed the first phase in the evolution of contemporary palliative care. I have argued that while this may characterize the beginning of modern palliative care it has evolved to adopt a less overtly Christian value base in favour of a communitarian model albeit deeply influenced by Christian values. Values such as the sanctity of life, the importance of death as an 'event' in life, and the family centred model of care that are regularly rehearsed and incorporated in official statements, strongly reflect this position. I offer this view as a *feasible* account in the knowledge that other interpretations are possible. It seems almost inevitable that the price of becoming a modern health speciality is secularization and with it an inexorable secularization of palliative care ethics requiring secular, rather than theological justification for its core values. This is not to say that justification is not possible, but rather that, to date, with the exception of Randall and Downie's contribution, most of those values remain largely unexamined axioms of palliative care.

One issue on which there is near universal agreement within palliative care is the acceptance of death, but the denial of a right to die. I shall go on to examine this argument in more detail. Viewed in the context of the history of palliative care and its underpinning Christian axiology, this stance against euthanasia and assisted dying seems to remain theological rather than philosophical in nature. Admittedly, it would be going too far to generalize the claim that the whole of modern palliative care shares the same specifically Christian proscription against voluntary euthanasia, clearly objections to euthanasia may have a secular basis, a point acknowledged by the palliative care community (Association of Palliative

Medicine 1993). My point is rather that, given the Christian influence on palliative care, it is reasonable to suppose that the origins of this position are under the same influence. The significance of this point is that, although autonomy is recognized within palliative care as an important component of respect for persons, the scope of autonomy is constrained by an over-arching axiology, which takes a broadly Christian view of the good life. It is against such a background, I suggest that the anti-euthanasia stance of palliative care is taken. However, if the evangelism of palliative care as a health speciality requires it to be secularized, one must question how defensible such a stance is. The imposition of a Christian axiology appears overly prescriptive and is open to challenge on the same grounds that medical paternalism has been challenged.

The alternative is for palliative care to turn to secular bioethics to support its stance against euthanasia and pro 'good death', this is beginning to happen. Bioethics offers a number of approaches. One approach argues that the principle of respect for autonomy requires a distinction between autonomy as a *liberty* claim and autonomy as a *rights* claim and thereby argues that respect for autonomy is best understood as a liberty claim carries no obligation to fulfil positive requests. The second, but as yet underdeveloped, approach turns to axiology and the claim that a good life requires a good death. To pursue this approach requires an account of the good death and an argument that a good death is achievable for all. These lines of argument conform to two possible general strategies, one bold and the other more modest in purpose. The bolder aim is that a core purpose of palliative care is the *prevention* of euthanasia, the more modest purpose sees palliative care merely as an *alternative* to euthanasia. My general point is that so far, if one can speak of the palliative care 'community' then this community has not clarified to which of these strategies it is committed. An important implication of the more modest strategy is the possibility of palliative care existing alongside 'euthanasia service;' a possibility to be explored in the final chapter.

One criticism of communitarian approaches is that they are inherently conservative and do not foster reflexivity and internal criticism. Kymlicka comments: 'No matter how deeply implicated we find ourselves in a social practice, we feel capable of questioning whether the practice is a valuable one'; something which the palliative care community must take to heart. My suggestion is that if palliative care seeks to offer a model of the good death that is achievable and not merely ideal, then it must acknowledge not only the acceptability of engineering the parameters of the good death, but the possibility, in some circumstances, of engineering, death itself.

5 | Respect for persons: a framework for palliative care

Introduction

As discussed in the previous chapter, the concept of autonomy has come to dominate health care ethics and with it or at least with the dominant theory of autonomy comes a particular ethical and political conception of value. Autonomy is also tied to a particular conception of what it is to be a morally significant entity — a person. This version of autonomy is also used to articulate the boundary of permissible intervention between one person and another. Health care and the relationship between patient and health professional in particular is one arena in which this concept has been influential. In Western medicine at least there is now a consensus on an ethic of patient autonomy in place of medical paternalism. In the analysis I have given of autonomy, particularly in the context of palliative care, I have attempted to paint a fuller picture of where autonomy sits within an account of the person. Thinking in this way attends not only to one's own 'rights', but relationships with others out of which grow obligations and duties. Because people stand in relationships with others, this adds a further tier of complexity, the relational aspect of autonomy. This chapter is concerned with spelling out the practical implications of the version of autonomy that I have argued is consistent with palliative care values.

So far I have discussed autonomy as a moral principle, the principle of respect for autonomy, but it is essentially a description of a *capacity*, the capacity to think and reflect, and decide for oneself. In order to understand the moral principle we must consider the moves that take us from an understanding of this capacity to a commitment to a principle of respect for such a capacity. Following on from my account of autonomy in the previous chapter, autonomy understood as a capacity, influences our understanding of the moral principle of respect for autonomy in the sense that it implies a right to choose for oneself. Understanding autonomy is important to our understanding of how we treat people with respect and is therefore crucial to our understanding of moral judgements. For example, should we distinguish between the different kinds of choice a person might make in terms of understanding our obligation to respect such choices?

Autonomy is sometimes seen to clash with welfare and this seems a particular problem in the health context because primarily health aims to promote a particular welfare good. Although such tensions arise in the rest of life, consider the young child who protests her preference for cake over vegetables at every meal. It seems right to balance her diet with both vegetables and, at least a little, cake, for while she may be an authority on what she *likes* she is by no means an authority on what is good for her. One could go further and say that it would be doing her a serious wrong not to see her through childhood well nourished. Moreover, a failure to educate her palate, so that she finds a varied diet acceptable, would deny her the sorts of healthy practises that are likely to sustain her as an adult. So, on this account, a certain level of interference in the life of another is consistent with respect for that person because in this example such interference can be seen as instrumental in the development of that person. Of course, while this approach may be appropriate for the young child, would the same be true if she were 6-, 12- or 20-years-old? Now one's feelings as a parent might incline you to conclude that you have just the same reasons to care for your child whether she is 2- or 20-years-old, but reflections on autonomy and the moral status of the person might require us to begin to distinguish a difference in the degree of justification we have for intervening in the life of a child over an adult. This conclusion, however, also raises some interesting questions about the nature and role of autonomy. Is autonomy a good thing in itself, or is autonomy valued because it is instrumental to some other valued end or ends? What are we showing respect for when we respect a person's autonomy? The examples I have given are perhaps reasonably straightforward because they contrast two extremes. However, in these examples of family relationships, one can see that it might be a difficult task to judge how much control to maintain or freedom to allow to a growing child. Even when the child reaches a point where, by convention, it is time to let go, as a parent it is hard to stand by and let them make their own mistakes. Most parents would probably feel justified in 'expressing' an opinion if they felt their child was making a mistake that could be avoided. This intimate family model is, of course, not a universal model of the family, but it does offer a kind of plausible model for how people interact more generally with others; that is where there is a more intimate relationship then questioning and challenging the other out of concern for their interests is part of that relationship. Of course, on the 'street' we proceed on the basis that the strangers we encounter are conducting their affairs with the same degree of autonomy as we are ourselves. However, we also encounter people in other intimate contexts, and the relationship between health professional and patient is one, where the relationship seems to fall somewhere in between the stranger and the intimate. The paternalism of medicine, that has now been broadly rejected, was modelled too much on the parent and child relationship. It now seems obvious that this is not the appropriate relationship between doctor and patient, even when the patient is a child.

We have seen from the previous discussion of axiology that subjective accounts of the good life have a strong intuitive and philosophical appeal. By subjective, I mean forms of evaluation, which focus on the quality of a person's experiences, their feelings of pleasure or satisfaction when their life is going well. The intuitive appeal of the subjective view is that we all know from our *own* experiences what we enjoy or take satisfaction in. In the context of palliative care, it is uncontroversial to take at face value what people say about their experiences and preferences, hence, the notion of a patient centred approach to care.

This approach is compatible with a broadly liberal moral framework, a framework that places a high value on the freedom from interference. Whereas such approaches are generally sceptical of any single conception of the good life, they are very tolerant of the different lives that people choose to live. Along with the liberal inclination to accept one or other of many subjective theories of the good life comes a greater emphasis on the importance of autonomy, since, if there is no authoritative theory of a good life, people should be free to choose their own way of living. I have argued in earlier chapters that this is a very restricted view of how autonomy fits into a complex shared morality.

The very notion of a *rational* pleasure seeker suggests the value of a capacity for deliberation to a life in which we make trade-offs between different kinds of pleasure and between different possible life plans, suggesting other, arguably more important components that cannot be reasonably described as 'pleasures'. If we take such rational deliberation as part of what we mean by autonomy, then it seems reasonable to suggest that autonomy is not simply instrumental, but also constitutive of a good life.

Reflecting on the nature of the good life raises still further issues, for example, if we ask whether an individual is, in fact, an authority with regard to their own good. This seems problematic even if we restrict the forms of good to pleasure alone. We can distinguish, for example, between what it *feels* like to enjoy a particular experience and *knowledge* about the sorts of thing that we might enjoy. While the former may be private and unique to me, the latter is not. So while the subjective view seems plausible in many ways, it has limited practical plausibility when thinking about how palliative care attempts to promote the good for the patient. Patient and professional working together come to examine the different possibilities for what might be better or worse for the patient, but working in an area where there is likely to be considerable uncertainty. Consider this example:

Jack's life has become overshadowed by pain due to an advanced cancer. From Jack's perspective he believes that having less pain would be a much better life than his current experience but he also believes that the only means of relieving his pain is in death. Jack therefore asks to be killed because although he would prefer to continue living with no, or much reduced, pain he believes that the only effective way of ending his pain is to end his life. Of course we are bound to accept that Jack is an authority on his pain but not necessarily an authority on what will bring about the state of affairs he desires. What will bring about this desired state of affairs is a question that is open to independent enquiry, after all Jack's own thoughts on the matter are too bleakly contrasted and he seems closed to the possibilities further treatment may offer him. A justified form of intervention in this case would be to challenge Jack, in a supportive way, in an attempt to persuade him to try different treatments as a less drastic means of achieving his goal.

This approach does not imply that the good life is consistent with having one's life directed by others, rather than directing one's own life. Although this may seem feasible in the context of health care where a doctor is much more likely to know or at least accurately predict what is best for me in terms of my health care needs than I am. This thought is counter-intuitive to the basic idea that respect for autonomy is a part of what is required to show respect to a person. However, the possibility that others may know better than me, what is good for me, forces us to consider what the proper influence of the other over me ought to be.

The 'Jack' example says something about how we can begin to understand what it is to show respect for others. It seems reasonable to take steps to persuade Jack to try different means of controlling his pain given that there is a shared view of the objective, namely, being pain free. For Jack, being killed is merely instrumental to being pain free, even if it would be self-defeating in terms of his interest in continuing to live. A different scenario in which Jack regards death as his objective gives a different analysis. In this case, even if Jack's pain could be controlled in a non-fatal way, it would not be true, no matter how we described the situation, that Jack's pain-free existence was a good life for Jack if what he wanted was an end to his life.

Even though we may believe that imposing this restriction on Jack's choice is an ethical limitation justly applied. It cannot be the case that, because we believe it is better to live one's life to its natural end, this becomes true for the person who is made to do so unwillingly. To believe so would be to confuse ethics with axiology. This is a particular challenge for palliative care. Even though a person's life might be considerably improved by adequate symptom control and social support, this cannot make the person value the rest of their life if what they want is to control their ending. However, accepting this limitation is not inconsistent with the belief that it is also right in the practice of palliative care to challenge someone to reconsider his or her decision, to take into account expert advice or try alternative options. This may be an important way of demonstrating that the professionals have respect for that person by showing they have not given up on that person too easily.

Our own view of the good life is open to challenge, improvement even, by taking into account the views of others. This, at least, suggests that there are grounds for engaging in a debate, at the level of both the individual and the collective, if only in an attempt to improve upon an uncertain view about what makes life go best. However, there are other more substantive reasons for intervening in the good life plan of an individual. In judging the goodness of a life we may also raise questions about the nature and type of preference pursued. It is not the mere formulation and then satisfaction of preferences that count in our judgements about the good life, but rather the nature of those preferences and their relationship to one another.

Take another example, I am referred to a pain specialist for symptom control for my neurological pain, but I refuse to consider taking the anti-depressant drugs she suggests because I believe this would show my pain to be 'in the mind'. I would prefer to be treated with morphine because I have read that morphine is the best drug for cancer-related pain. What I choose on the basis of my fear and lack of knowledge will restrict the quality of life that I also strongly wish to enjoy; yet the doctor knows that I am likely to achieve this only if I accept the treatment. While we both agree on the goal, we disagree on the way to achieve it. It is possible therefore to judge, at least in some aspects, of what is good for a person from an objective perspective. This said, one must be cautious not to interpret this as an argument justi-fying the *imposition* of the treatment, although acknowledging the possi-bility of an objective perspective is the beginning of an argument about what constitutes justified intervention in the life of another person.

Between people there will always be differences of opinion about the relative value and importance of alternative life-styles that will not be resolved by appeal to objective qualities. People do have varied views and beliefs, and different ideas, about what constitutes a good life when seen as a whole, but at the same time, this does not require us to accept that such beliefs and plans could not be revised and improved upon. There is a danger, however, of confusing an ideology of the good life with particular strategies and interventions aimed at achieving a particular good. So, in palliative care, the ideology of the good death is an ideal that should be seen as quite distinct from the particular proven expertise that palliative care has for managing particular problems.

I believe that the version of the principle of respect for autonomy I have sketched here is compatible with the practice of palliative care. In my view, respect for autonomy requires that we weigh carefully the reasons for constraining the wishes of another or otherwise intervening in their life. Good reasons may justify such intrusions, even at times against the wishes of the individual concerned. However, a note of caution, what I have in mind here for the palliative care context are interventions such as directing, guiding, even coercing a person in their interests, where there are the strongest reasons for doing so and the probability of achieving the goal is high. Here, I have in mind an example where a person is in chronic pain and wishes to be pain free, but does not wish to take opiates, then he might be strongly persuaded to try such a drug.

However, this view also requires that we ought to defer authority to the individual on questions of their own good, and support robustly a right of non-interference when the degree of uncertainty as to the good of the outcome is high. In other words, we may be agnostic as to whether there is an authority with regard to what is good in a particular instance, in which case, to be consistent with the version of autonomy I am espousing, priority should be given to the views of the individual whose life it is. In the final chapter, I shall discuss a particular implication of this position for end-of-life choices.

An ethical framework: autonomy in practice

In this section I want to explore how the principle of respect for autonomy, as I have outlined it, can be applied in practice. The application will follow the categories of an ethical framework illustrated in Figure 5.1.

Figure 5.1 Categories of an ethical framework

Best Interests	• Objective • Subjective • Absolute
Wishes, choices, preferences	• Wishes/choices • Other Interests
Family concerns	• Nature of • Authority of
Other regarding	• Political • Legal • Social

(Reprinted with permission from Woods (2005)

Consider the following case.

Helen, a 58-year-old retired biology teacher, who has lived with Multiple Sclerosis (MS) for 25 years. For the past 10 years, Helen has been confined to a wheelchair and is heavily dependent upon physical care. She is now taking a very soft or liquid diet and finds it harder to swallow. Helen says that she now takes no pleasure in eating whatsoever. Following a spate of recent hospital admissions for dehydration, secondary to a bladder infection, she has decided that she will not go into hospital again. Helen has appeared rather low in mood but not overtly depressed, and is pleasant to her family, visiting nurses and carers. She lives with her husband and their two daughters live nearby.

Helen asks to see her physician, as she wishes to make it clear that she has reached a decision. She says that she believes that she has come to the end of what she regards to be a worthwhile life and has no wish to prolong things. She feels that she has said all that needs to be said to her family and friends. Helen knows that she cannot ask for euthanasia as such, but now intends to stop drinking in order to hasten her death herself. She wants to know that she *can* do this, that she will be kept comfortable and that no one will set up an intravenous infusion when she cannot argue with them.

The next day, her husband and one of her daughters wish to speak to someone. They are unhappy about Helen's decision, and request a subcutaneous drip, an intervention used several times in the past. This, they suggest, is to be started immediately or if she becomes too weak to say 'no'. The other daughter is apparently 'siding with her mother'.

By reflecting on this case and using other examples, I will now give an account of how the principle of respect for autonomy might be applied in practice, taking each category of the moral framework in turn.

Best interests

In the health care context, health professionals commonly talk of 'best interests', often as a justification for, but also as the aim of certain kinds of intervention. A person's 'best interests' could be defined in terms of the particular good that health care interventions aim for. In other words, 'best interests' seem to be a claim about an objective good, but is this all 'best interests' means? On reflection there seems to be at least three significant components to best interests and it is worthwhile attempting to distinguish these.

First, there is the version of best interests most commonly intended by health professionals, namely the person's objective health interests. Now, it is certainly the case that an *objective* best interests argument can often provide the strongest reasons for intervening in the life of another person even where that person has different ideas about what is in their interests, but mindful that 'best objective health interests' is a very restricted sense of best interests when compared with someone's overall interests. Perhaps the clearest example of an application of the objective' best interests' argument is with a victim of a road accident, where the seriously-injured driver insists that she is fine and does not wish to be taken to hospital, although it is clear she has very serious injuries. In this case, it would seem right for the health professionals at the scene to disregard the patient's view and take her to hospital. Imagine that, by the time the trauma victim arrives at the hospital, she has become unconscious and has lost a lot of blood, it would seem reasonable to stop the bleeding and make good the blood loss.

A less dramatic example is the patient who visits his doctor because of a heavy cold. The patient feels awful and wants something to make him feel better. He expects the doctor to prescribe antibiotics. The doctor, however, argues that antibiotics will have no effect on the cold virus and advises the patient to take palliative measures, whilst reassuring him that if he does not feel better soon he can return to the surgery. However, the patient is not happy; he insists that he has had antibiotics in the past for similar ailments and he wants the same treatment now.

In this situation, the doctor's continuing refusal to give the patient what he wants seems justified since viruses do not respond to such treatment. Moreover, to give antibiotics would be to risk an important common good, a good in which this patient would no doubt also wish to partake, namely the availability of a range of effective antibiotics for the treatment of bacterial infections. Now these two cases seem relatively clear examples of where the notion of best interests can be understood as *best* objective health interests, and it seems reasonable to allow the degree of intrusiveness and constraint on the other's wishes that the health professional's judgement entails. The health professional's judgement carries both epistemic and moral weight because there is a fact of the matter about which the doctor has best evidence and the doctor employs this evidence within a valid moral judgement. Difficulties arise when the relative importance of such objective interests are called into question. Reflecting on the case of Helen, it could be argued that in terms of her *objective* health interests, she would benefit from some form of feeding and certainly from being adequately hydrated, she would probably feel more comfortable and perhaps even live longer. However, what is called into question in this instance is the priority that should be given to these objective health interests when weighed against the other interests Helen has with regard to her own death.

When reflecting on the reasons one may give in favour of intervening in the life of another, weight must be given to a person's interests as seen from their perspective; their *subjective* interests. To say an interest is subjective is not to say that it is *private*, in the sense that only the person whose interests we are discussing can know about it. The subjective view is merely the view of a person's interests as seen from the 'inside' so to speak, from the perspective of *this* person. Such a view is private only in the sense that others can only usually gain insight into this perspective when the person reveals it to them. Now in terms of what weight the subjective view carries in determining a person's best interests it would seem that where a person is capable of having such a view it ought to be given at least equal weight to that of the objective view. Where there is uncertainty about what is in a persons overall best interests, and I would suggest that this is most cases, it would seem reasonable to give *more* weight to the subjective view, since if there is a mistake to be made, it is better that a person makes their own mistakes than has the mistakes of others forced upon them. This is not to say that the subjective view isn't open to challenge. A person can be challenged morally or intellectually by pointing to deficits in their reasoning, their factual knowledge or by presenting them, through argument and discussion, with an alternative view.

To complete this taxonomy of interests, there is the category I describe as *absolute* interests. The term 'absolute' is not meant in any strict sense, but rather to represent those interests, whatever they are, which represent what that individual sees as central to their identity. Where a decision to intervene or not in the life of another rests on the balance of interests, then such interests can be played as the most powerful 'trump card' against the other sorts of interests that can be mustered together as reasons for intervening. For example, a Roman Catholic woman is informed that she is 12 weeks pregnant with her much wanted first pregnancy, but that she also has an advanced tumour of the cervix that can only be effectively treated by hysterectomy. Her faith in God and her belief in the sanctity of life of her unborn child means that she cannot consent to a treatment that would result in the death of her child. The woman insists upon her decision, even though her Church may sanction such an action under these circumstances, and failure to take any action threatens her own life and the life of the child. Now her position begins to take on the status of an absolute interest in so far as we can be satisfied that she has been made aware of the other reasons for intervening in this situation and the likely consequences of her action. If, in the light of such a discussion, the woman feels that life would be intolerable lived in the shadow of such a decision then there is a point at which such a view ought not to be overridden. The weight of absolute interests has been long recognized where certain religious convictions have led to the refusal of a life-saving intervention such as a blood transfusion. However, absolute interests do not have to be grounded in religious faith, any sincere conviction held in the face of the other reasons for intervening should be afforded such moral weight. Of course, the term 'absolute' interest is something of a metaphor, a way of giving weight to a person's interests and values where the consequences of abiding by these are severe for the person whose interests they are. Helen's refusal of nutrition and hydration might be regarded as an expression of an absolute interest, her only means of having the control over her end, where more direct methods are denied her. Some members of her family have difficulty accepting this decision, believing they have the right to override such a decision. However, their reasons are *theirs* and, as such, do not weigh against Helen's judgement. On paper, this is an easy analysis to make, but palliative care workers may find themselves attempting to support both Helen and her family at a time of acute emotion. There is a further duty on palliative care workers to find a means of supporting both Helen and her family in a way that respects Helen's decision, and gently, but firmly remind the family of the constraints on their right to intrude.

Wishes, preferences, choices

There is clearly some overlap here with the previous category, but there are also some important differences. Before going on to explore these differences I want to say something about why there should be such a category as wishes, choices and preferences in the framework when some might argue, although I believe wrongly, that this category could be adequately described by one word — 'autonomy'.

One of the difficulties with the concept of autonomy is the common use of the term combined with its complexity of meaning. Autonomy has now become an accepted shorthand in circumstances that really require a great deal more conceptual 'unpacking'. Take, for example, the fact that autonomy has at least two distinct uses, not always distinguished in practice. One is autonomy as a capacity and the other is autonomy as a moral principle. The definition of autonomy as a capacity for making reflective choices is important, since it is seen by some as a sufficient condition for a certain kind of moral status. Having such a capacity is merely a starting point in the sense that the exercise of this capacity is dependent on further conditions, some of which are intrinsic to the individual and some of which are extrinsic. Intrinsic conditions include, at the very basic level, a functioning brain, but also a certain level of cognitive capacity, which would include such things as memory, imagination and the capacity to assimilate knowledge. Extrinsic conditions include the environment and freedom to act, for example. Perhaps the single most important extrinsic factor for autonomy is *relational* in that the extent to which one can expect one's own autonomy to be respected is relative to the right and freedom of others to act autonomously. This implies a number of things; my autonomy is enhanced by and dependent upon others in that I might rely on them as a source of information, or as manipulators of the environment or as other actors, who may permit or constrain my own actions. These conditions of autonomy are very obvious in palliative care. The woman with advanced disease, confined to bed and with little movement in her limbs is denied the most ordinary freedom if the remote control for the TV is too far away, her drinking glass empty and her attendant call-device beyond her reach. The man whose cancer has recurred relies upon the doctor for information if he is to decide to enter a phase one clinical trial of a new cancer drug. The woman with advancing neurological disease who asks her doctor for a prescription of a lethal cocktail of drugs so that she may end her life at a moment of her own choosing, encroaches on the autonomy of the person to whom she makes the request.

Attempting to elicit and, indeed, attending to a person's wishes, choices and preferences are means of gaining insight into their interests. Giving moral weight to a person's interests is a statement about the place the individual has in shaping and directing his or her own life. This goes some way to describing a principle of respect for persons that accommodates a principle of respect for autonomy. We may consider it important to respect a person's wishes, even though they may lack autonomy and, indeed, be dead. However, what flows from this is relative to the obligations and autonomy of others. Nor does it mean that we should always and everywhere give people what they wish, choose or prefer or even accept such things at face value. Your own view of your own good may be improved from the 'outside', so to speak, by being challenged by alternative views.

Wishes may range from aspirations for the possible, the *improbable* to the *impossible* and can be regarded as intensely personal, if not private. It would seem overly intrusive to suggest that a person's wishes, in so far as they are a feature of that person's mental life, ought to be constrained in any way. However, where wishes give rise to concrete choices, then wishes ought to be influenced in a number of ways, including what might be termed a 'reality constraint'. For example, the sort of information given to the patient considering participating in a clinical trial should focus on the probable, rather than the improbable, even though the individual's decision may in part be influenced by a desire for the improbable.

A task in palliative care may be to challenge and change even a person's preferences, where these are based on deficient or even false knowledge, or so limiting as to be easily improved upon, as Rebecca Dresser remarks:

> We do not advance people's autonomy by giving effect to choices that originate in insufficient or mistaken information. Indeed interference in such choices is often considered a form of justified paternalism.
>
> (Dresser 1995: 35)

Although, as a general rule, there is good reason to set the threshold for capacity at the lowest possible level, so as to include as many individuals as possible into the class of decision makers, there is also a good reason to be discerning between different sorts of decision. Forms of justified intervention that the palliative care worker might consider, include a formal assessment of the capacity of the person to make the decision they now wish to make (Grisso and Appelbaum 1998), although it might be too easy to declare an unpopular decision 'incompetent'. More usual interventions would include informing the person of relevant facts and exploring the possible alternatives with them. In extreme cases, and Helen's situation may be regarded as such, then confronting the decision maker with the likely consequences of their decision both for themselves and for those close to them might be justified. In my view, such measures could be regarded as a means of acknowledging both Helen's autonomy and her responsibility. In this respect, although we may regard Helen's decision to stop eating and drinking as justified in relation to her 'absolute' interest in controlling her end-of-life choices, we may also regard, as part of our respect for Helen as a person, a need to explore with her the likely impact of such a decision on those who are close to her.

The family

In each category discussed so far, I have attempted to sketch an account of the extent and scope of individual autonomy, describing as it were the boundary conditions of individual autonomy. One set of conditions involves the individual's own capacities and also the environment in which they are located, another involves relational factors. Among these, the family is often singled out as constituting a special network of meaningful relationships. In the context of health care, the family represents another layer of complexity in the decision-making process. Health workers frequently encounter the family of patients who, by virtue of their status as family, assume a 'right' to be taken into confidence, sometimes claiming the authority to be involved in making decisions for the patient. It is understandable that such an assumption might be borne out of their intimacy with the patient. After all, a person who is close to the patient may be more successful in their speculation about what is in the interests of an incompetent person rather than the health professional who is a stranger. Indeed, the family may as Blustein suggests 'shore up the patient's vulnerable autonomy' (Blustein 1993: 6). To do justice to family relationships it has been argued that, rather than an ethics of strangers, an ethics of intimates should be applied. Weijer (2000) argues that it is strange to apply a principle of confidentiality, for example, to families who already share an 'indissoluble bond'. However, we do have reason to be at least a little circumspect about what we mean by the family relationship and what follows morally from such a relationship. First, how is 'family' to be defined? The idea of a man and woman who are married with children is but one form of family relationship that, in a pluralistic society, might also include unmarried partners, same-sex couples or any combination of such relationships deemed 'significant' by those involved in them. I doubt, however, that any such relationship constitutes an indissoluble bond in any significant moral sense of that term. What matters in the palliative care context, where there are likely to be complex decisions to be made, is that every effort is made to identify the 'significant other' at the earliest opportunity.

Having raised doubts about there being any necessary form of family, we must also be cautious about what follows, in circumstances where it has been possible to establish the fact of such a relationship. Take the claim about confidentiality, for example. We may accept the point that families do have intimate knowledge of one another, but still acknowledge that, even within families, there is usually a line drawn between what is and is not common family knowledge. Take, for example, the fact that my wife keeps a diary. Although I am close to her and know many personal things about her, it does not follow that I am entitled to read her diary without her permission. In the context of patient/family relationships, the palliative care worker must act as an honest broker when dealing with the sometimes conflicting claims of family members. Consider the man who has six sisters all who love him dearly. However, if he lay in a coma surrounded by his sisters then there would be at least six different points of view about what was best for him. The telling point is that perhaps none of these views would coincide with what he would want for himself! So while we may have a strong intuition that the family has a role in determining a person's best interests, it cannot be a unique or privileged view.

Nothing hinges, morally speaking, on the 'family' as a unique institution, but this is not to say that that there are no special relationships, including more conventional notions of family, between people and groups of people. Nor is this to say that the criticisms levelled at respect for autonomy in the context of families are misplaced. However, by treading cautiously it is possible to see what is important about *individual* autonomy without, at the same time, downgrading the importance of family or other significant relationships between people.

Respect for autonomy is perhaps too abstract a concept for significant others to consider when their focus is caring for their loved one, but if it is necessary to defend individual autonomy, even within the context of a loving family relationship, then palliative care workers can employ practical strategies rather than elaborate moral arguments to secure this goal. To employ a policy of open communication, with the patient and family members, the health professional must first establish the patient's preferences for sharing information about their condition and prognosis. While some patients welcome open and honest communication between their professional carers, themselves and their family; some do not and, therefore, it would be as wrong to assume this as to deny that the family should be informed. Real life complexity requires prior groundwork to determine preferences of this kind and the flexibility to respond to changing circumstances. Palliative care workers ought to encourage patients, not just to express their preferences, but also to think about the consequences of having their preferences met. This is one context in which talk of the correlative responsibility alongside the rights of autonomy can be seen. The patient who refuses to disclose their condition to the family in order to protect them ought to be made aware of what is likely to follow from their decision.

Other regarding

The family is but one example of where there are important other regarding constraints upon individual autonomy. To consider a proper view of the individual and their rights, one must consider how we understand the very concept of the individual. We have spent some time criticizing the highly abstract interpretation of autonomy, advanced by some liberals, which sees the person as a unique individual isolated from any context and divorced of relationships. There are important justified constraints on what the patient can demand, just as there are such constraints on what the health professional is obliged or ought to do.

What a patient may request of a health professional is necessarily constrained because what the health professional can do is circumscribed by their professional and legal duties. For example, many practitioners may find themselves able to agree with, and perhaps even support Helen's decision to stop eating and drinking. However, I believe most palliative care workers would find it problematic if she had requested a lethal injection or advice on how to hurry her end still further. I am not offering the conservative argument that laws and guidelines should not be challenged. I am suggesting that, although the relationship between health professional and patient is privileged, it is so within a broader context of constraint — professional, legal and social in nature. Those who might be sympathetic with a request for euthanasia from Helen should seek to change the law prohibiting such acts by democratic means, rather than by dramatic individual gestures. Individuals are also constrained by social values and the personal values of others. Indeed, as I have argued, the grounds of an individual's autonomy requires a margin of reciprocity and tolerance for the autonomy of others.

Finally, there are considerations of justice and distributive justice in particular in which the rights and claims of an individual must be weighed against the claims of others. Balancing the claims of different individuals may necessitate constraints on what people claim for themselves. At the macro-level of government, balancing the sometimes competing interests of different people and determining the set of compromises that can best provide for such interests is the proper role of government (Dworkin 1993). In other words a condition of living within a society entails that we submit to some constraints on our autonomy in order to enjoy the benefits of that society. The same is also true of the micro-level of individual patient decisions where health professionals have an equally legitimate role in balancing the competing interests of different individuals even as to how a doctor or nurse divides her time between the demanding and vociferous patient, for example, and, the much sicker, but silent other. Respect for the autonomy of individual patients is necessarily constrained by what I have described as 'other regarding' considerations.

Conclusion

In this chapter and the previous one, I have moved from an account of the contemporary meaning of autonomy, and how this has been influenced by various philosophical and political ideas, to a practical model of how a principle of respect for autonomy can be applied to palliative care. The ethical framework I describe is but one form of device practitioners may use to aid reflection on the reasons underpinning their judgements to intervene, or not, in the lives of their patients. This chapter is not the place to reflect on the intricacies of effective communication and emotional support, although these are also necessary elements in a complete reflective framework.

Palliative care is one discipline within health care that has a strong view as to the nature of the good it aims to promote in terminal disease. The good or goods of palliative care have quite diverse origins from religious, and specifically Christian, influences to the liberal secular ethics, and the communitarian model described in the previous chapter. What I have argued in this chapter is that, although it seems implausible that there can be an absolute authority as to the nature of the good life for individuals, it is not so implausible that certain goods can be established objectively. Candidates for such goods in the context of palliative care would no doubt include being pain-free, but might also include such values as dignity, reconciliation and peaceful death, all elements of the 'good death'. However, advocates of such 'objective' goods must be mindful of the phenomenon of 'endorsement constraint' as an important limiting factor (Dworkin 1989). What this means is that, although we might convince people to conform to a set of values, say for example, to a palliative care ideal of 'good death', mere conformity cannot make a person's life go better from the subjective perspective. A crucial question in applying a principle of respect for autonomy, therefore, is under what circumstances or for what reasons do we give weight to that subjective perspective?

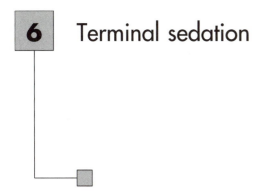

6 Terminal sedation

Introduction

'Terminal Sedation' (TS) is an emotive phrase and in this chapter I will discuss the role and purpose of sedation at the end of life with a view to spanning the breadth of its application from its least controversial, as an adjunct to symptom control, to its most controversial application in the terminal phase of dying. The 1990 report by Ventafridda *et al.* pointed to the significant role that sedation plays in the control of a number of common refractory symptoms (symptoms unresponsive to standard treatment) at the end of life. Although the frequency of the use of sedation has been contested, there is general agreement that sedation is a necessary intervention in terminal care (Chernoy and Portenoy 1994; Porta Sales 2001; Broeckaert and Nunez-Olarte 2002). The variations in protocol, criteria for use and range of substances used have been frequently reported and debated. Some of the most heated debate has concerned the use of sedation in a context not usually associated with palliative care, such as the withdrawal of ventilation, but it has also been widely discussed in the context of withdrawing artificial nutrition and hydration (Billings and Block 1996; Brody 1996; Quill and Brock 2000; Quill *et al.* 2000).

The ethical issues associated with sedation or, more specifically, terminal sedation in palliative care were crystallized by Materstvedt and Kaasa (2000) and Tännsjö (2000, 2004). In this chapter, I shall begin by considering Tännsjö's analysis of TS and his recommendation that TS offers an alternative form of end-of-life treatment for those who hold a principled objection to euthanasia. In this chapter, I will consider the arguments both for and against Tännsjö's position. I shall go on to argue that TS, as a term, should be abandoned in favour of *palliative* sedation and I shall go on to show that, as a form of treatment, palliative sedation is a legitimate intervention entirely compatible with the principles of good palliative care at the end-of-life.

While debates about terminal and palliative sedation have been conducted since the early 1990s, the definition of the term *palliative* sedation, discussion of its appropriate application and ethical aspects, has only more recently appeared in the professional journals. In a personal communication with Lars Johan Matersvedt, he informs me that it was probably his publication with Stein Kaasa (Matersvedt and Kaasa 2000) in which the term was first defined in print. Matersvedt and Kaasa's definition was subsequently adopted by the Norwegian Medical Association. In December 2000, Bert Broeckaert offered his own definition of palliative sedation in an abstract at the first European Association of Palliative Care (subsequently published as Broeckaert 2002). In developing my argument in support of palliative sedation I draw on these and other sources.

Terminal sedation: Tännsjö's position

Tännsjö's analysis of TS was inspired by a number of clinical cases much discussed in Sweden in 1996 and 1997. It was based on the practises in these cases that Tännsjö developed his definition of terminal sedation (TS), which reads:

> ... a procedure where through heavy sedation a terminally ill patient is put into a state of coma, where the intention of the doctor is that the patient should stay comatose until he or she is dead. No extraordinary monitoring of the medical state of the patient is undertaken. Normal hydration is ignored. All this means that in certain cases where patients are being terminally sedated, death is hastened; if the disease does not kill the patient, some complication in relation to the sedation, or the withdrawal of treatment and hydration, or the combination of these, does.
>
> (Tännsjö 2004: 15)

Reviewing the debate that has been ongoing since the 1990s, Tännsjö suggests that there are three discernible positions. The first position regards TS as always wrong, and this is the view associated most closely with the issue of sedating patients prior to their removal from artificial ventilation (Troug *et al.* 1991). The second takes the view that TS is an intervention of a last resort, when all other efforts to control symptoms have failed and it is impossible to use anything less than heavy sedation (Dunlop *et al.* 1995). The third position regards TS as one option among many and should be provided at the patient's request in the face of refractory symptoms (Lawrence and Schneiderman 1991).

Tännsjö's stance, as implied from his definition of TS, is consistent with the third position. Tännsjö defends this position and also advocates the use of TS by arguing that even though TS may contribute to the death of the patient, it is distinct from forbidden forms of killing (forbidden in most countries), such as euthanasia. Tännsjö develops his argument by showing how TS sits with the standard forms of argument used to distinguish morally and legally accepted forms of killing from the forms of killing that are mostly forbidden.

The distinction rests upon the two traditional forms of argument, the acts and omissions distinction, and the doctrine of double effect. Although these arguments have been much criticized, they nevertheless continue to underpin traditional ethical and legal arguments in this context. Tännsjö suggests that it is necessary to rehearse these arguments because he believes that they can be shown to be clear, valid and compatible with standard medical ethical practises they render the sorts of distinction outlined in the table shown in Figure 6.1 cogent and defensible.

Figure 6.1   Categories of killing

FORMS of KILLING	Death is intended	Death is merely foreseen
Active forms	FORBIDDEN	TOLERATED
Passive forms	TOLERATED	TOLERATED

(Adapted with permission from Tännsjö 2004: 19.)

Tännsjö's first task is to deal with the much criticized distinction between acts and omissions. Tännsjö considers this to be a valid distinction because we can and, more importantly, do distinguish between active and passive actions. Tännsjö tells us that it is always wrong, for example, to kill actively, but passive killing may sometimes be acceptable. He accepts that in the case of particular actions it may sometimes be difficult to categorize absolutely an action as either passive or active, since particular actions can admit to being either passive or active descriptions. However, he argues that certain kinds of action admit to being sorted into active or passive instances. To illustrate the point, Tännsjö uses the example of 'helping', of which there may be passive instances or active instances, and he argues that 'killing' is but another example of this kind of action. There can be 'active' killing and there can be 'passive' killing (letting nature take its course). Although there can be no absolute criterion to distinguish active from passive, it is possible to formulate good enough reasons to support our intuitions that a particular action falls into one category, rather than another. Tännsjö concludes, however, that the active/passive or acts and omissions distinction is, taken alone, not a distinction that has great ethical force in medicine, as both forms of killing are regarded as ethical and legal in some circumstances (Tännsjö 2004: 18).

However, Tännsjö argues that, when it comes to the doctrine of double effect, then the traditional interpretation of this principle says that it is always wrong intentionally to kill; a view that is readily advanced by the palliative care community. It may be ethical to kill or hasten the end of a patient provided that their death is merely foreseen, but not directly intended. Acts in which this occurs must have the principal aim of doing good, by a means that is itself proportionate to the intended good. Tännsjö then goes on to point out that, although the distinction may be clear and valid, most western countries do not abide by it either, as the many cases of withdrawing and withholding life-sustaining treatment from incompetent patients illustrates. Tännsjö's point is that only a combination of the two principles can defend the traditional objection to euthanasia, and with the exception of Belgium and the Netherlands, this is the position reflected in most western jurisdictions. This is the position located in the top left-hand section of the figure, which illustrates that the combination of active intentional killing is forbidden. This is also, Tännsjö contends, the position endorsed by supporters of the Sanctity-of-life Doctrine.

This digression by Tännsjö is justified because, although he is neither a supporter of these principles nor the Sanctity-of-life Doctrine, he wishes to explore their implications for his version of TS. Tännsjö is candid that such a defence of TS should mean that TS is an acceptable practice in a context in which euthanasia is condemned.

This is how Tännsjö sees TS fitting with the traditional approach: sedation may cause death, but sedation does not aim at death, only at palliating symptoms, with the awareness that death may be an unintended side-effect. Therefore, even if sedation actively kills the patient this is not intended and so falls outside of the forbidden category. This is how Randall and Downie justify the use of sedation in their 1999 book:

> In situations of severe distress such as mental anguish, restlessness, or unrelieved pain, autonomous patients may ask for or be offered sedation. This is given with the intention of alleviating distress ... However if distress is so severe as to require greater sedation if it is to be relieved, then there is a significant risk that life may be shortened ... The benefit of alleviating severe distress is considered by patients and carers to outweigh the possible harm by shortening the duration of the terminal illness. Sedation sufficient to alleviate distress is used. Intentional overdoses of either analgesics or sedative medication are not morally justified.
>
> (Randall and Downie 1999: 119)

This is one of the clearest statements of the application of the principle of double effect in the context of terminal care and it is well worth pondering the detail of this statement. The options are these: give less sedation than will relieve the patient of the level of distress they find intolerable or give greater sedation with some uncertain risk of shortening life. The latter part of the previous sentence 'shortening life' I take to be an acceptable substitution for the expression 'shortening the duration of the terminal illness'. This must be an acceptable and, indeed, uncontroversial substitution, since how else are we to understand terminal illness? 'Shortening life' and 'shortening the course of the terminal illness' can therefore be substituted one for the other without changing the meaning of the sentence.

It should also be noted that Randall and Downie utilize an additional ethical argument; evident in this quotation. This argument draws upon a different moral tradition than the doctrines I have been describing. It is the argument that weighs the benefits against the risks and is therefore a consequentialist form of argument, and is one method of judging the proportionality of an intervention. In their 2006 book Randall and Downie state their position unambiguously:

> Health care practitioners may justifiably hasten death as a foreseen but not intended effect of treatment whose aim is the relief of pain and distress at the end of life ... In the philosophy of palliative care, as in health care ethics and the law generally, letting die must be permitted. Letting die here means withholding or withdrawing a life-prolonging treatment when its harms and risks exceeds its benefits. Health care practitioners who act in this way neither intend nor cause the patient's death.
>
> (Randall and Downie 2006: 221)

I cite both quotations, because as exemplars of the contemporary palliative care approach, they are consistent with Tännsjö's schema. However, Randall and Downie show this position to be inconsistent with the WHO (2002) statement, which says that palliative care 'intends neither to hasten nor postpone death'. Taken at face value this does potentially conflict with the acceptance of TS.

Some problems with Tännsjö's account and an alternative approach

Helga Khuse and others (Tännsjö 2004) have contended that Tännsjö's attempt to render his version of TS compatible with the views of the supporters of the Sanctity-of-Life Doctrine is flawed. Moreover, Tännsjö's position on TS is, in fact, merely a Trojan horse for euthanasia. I will now consider some of the criticisms levelled at Tännsjö's account of TS as a way of clarifying some of the conceptual issues associated with TS before turning to an account of sedation within palliative care that meets some of these objections.

First, I shall say something about why it is necessary to think about approaches to treatment in terms of their underlying ethical justification rather than by merely asserting a protocol based upon 'evidence'. In chapter 3, I argued that, in so far as it can be made explicit, the ethical stance of the hospice movement rested firmly within Christian moral ethos. Catholic and protestant orders were the founders of homes for the dying and acted in fulfilment of Christian duty. The practises of care were driven by belief in the sanctity of life and a traditional Christian *ars moriendi* view of death and dying. These values became more overtly expressed, most clearly so, in the writings of Cicely Saunders. I have also argued that in the evolution of palliative care, from the modern hospice movement in parallel with the more explicit discussion of values and ethics, there was also a secular shift in values. This secular shift might be seen to have a number of drivers including the increasing diversity and secularization of society, making an exclusively Christian approach inappropriate. During this time, the role of doctors became more important. With the acceptance of palliative medicine as a medical speciality, Doctors became a central force behind evolving palliative care practises. With the increased role for medicine there also came the pressure for palliative care to adopt the ethical approach increasingly dominant within medicine, a secular liberal approach to ethics. However, I have also argued that, within the palliative care community's open discussion of ethics and values, there is a resistance to liberal approaches, expressed implicitly, as a form of communitarian ethics. However, the pressure to adopt liberal ethics is still evident in the move for palliative care to abandon its claim to distinctiveness from other health disciplines. The communitarian approach does offer a means of articulating the distinctiveness of palliative care. I suggest that the articulation of a communitarian philosophy offers a vehicle for expressing a secular version of *ars moriendi*, which may prove a powerful means of maintaining the distinctiveness of palliative care. The account of palliative sedation I develop in this chapter is an example of how such an approach may be brought to bear on practice. To develop this approach it is necessary to first consider Tännsjö's account of TS.

As I have argued, the belief in the sanctity of life has had a strong influence upon palliative care. The Sanctity-of-Life Doctrine has its origins in Judaeo-Christian thought and is concerned with the absolute prohibition on the taking of innocent life. The basic premise upon which this position is based is that human life is a gift from God and, therefore, it is not within the gift of humankind to take an innocent life even one's own. As Kuhse rightly points out, although many people no longer subscribe to traditional religious doctrines, the Sanctity-of-Life Doctrine has without question informed normative values and legal principles (Kuhse 2004: 59). This does not quite sit with Tännsjö's account in which he argues that the Sanctity-of-Life Doctrine is compatible with intentional passive killing, the lower left category of the table (Figure 6.1).

The prohibition on intentional passive killing is echoed in the Vatican's

Declaration on Euthanasia, which defines euthanasia/mercy killing as 'an action or an omission which of itself or by intention causes death' (Sacred Congregation for the Doctrine of the Faith 1980: 6). Stated in this way the Sanctity-of-Life Doctrine seems unambiguous in its position. However, it must also be added that supporters of this position also accept that there is no obligation to do everything possible to prolong life. Where such decisions do not involve the intentional ending of a life then it is regarded as permissible to withhold or withdraw 'extraordinary' or disproportionate treatment, or administer treatment which may unintentionally shorten life (1980: 8–9). On this point it would appear that Helga Kuhse's analysis of Tännsjö's argument is correct, the Sanctity-of-Life Doctrine does not accept as permissible the category of intentional passive killing (Kuhse 2004: 60).

However, the idea of intentional passive killing has become broadly accepted within western medicine, even and especially, within contexts where there is an explicit rejection of euthanasia (Materstvedt *et al.* 2003). I suggest that the acceptability of this position is indicative of the 'secular shift' in contemporary medical ethics and, since the ethics of palliative care have undergone a similar shift, then, intentional passive killing ought to be (and indeed is) acceptable to palliative care, although some may object to this particular phraseology. The traditional Sanctity-of-Life Doctrine ought to be regarded as a particular view of some religious groups, but not as representative of the secular ethical norms of medicine. I believe that the strength of Tännsjö's argument is to make a robust defence of this position but that he is mistaken, and Kuhse is correct to claim that this is *not* a position compatible with the Sanctity-of-Life Doctrine. However, several important questions remain: is TS a form of intentional passive killing, and is it consistent to accept intentional passive killing yet maintain an objection to euthanasia? It is these questions that this and the next chapter will address.

Terminal sedation/palliative sedation: an alternative model

Although I contend that TS can be distinguished from euthanasia TS does raise questions concerning the nature of the good death and what constitutes good care at the end of life. I now argue that the acceptability of TS within palliative care and the distinction between TS and euthanasia requires a more careful definition. Here, I shall argue for the integration of Tännsjö's account of TS into a broader concept of, *palliative* sedation (PS) as it has been defined by Materstvedt and Kaasa (2000) and Broeckaert (2000). The justification for using terminal sedation, I shall argue, requires a more nuanced awareness to the spectrum of circumstances in which sedation is utilized within palliative care. A key feature of the justification for the use of PS requires a separation of decisions to use PS from other end-of-life treatment decisions; the withdrawal or withholding of artificial hydration and nutrition in particular.

Palliative care at the end-of-life

Chapter 2 identified the development of the modern palliative care movement as having its origins in a number of pioneering events and individuals. In the UK, palliative care emerged from the early hospice movement (Clark and Seymour 1999). Hospice philosophy was defined and developed from the 1950s onwards by Cicely Saunders among others. Working and writing as a nurse, Saunders was one of the first scholars to set out the basic principles of the care for the dying: 'Care for the dying person should be directed no longer towards his cure, rehabilitation or even palliation but primarily at his comfort' (1966: 225). It was the emphasis on comfort and care that was the inspiration for many health workers to work with the dying who they believed had been abandoned by mainstream healthcare (Woods 2001). Care of the dying, until the advent of palliative medicine in 1987, was predominantly a nursing domain with hospices being run by nurses; usually calling upon the services of a sympathetic local doctor for support. Therefore, 'medical' interventions were minimal and nursing care was the mainstay of hospice care. The recognition of palliative medicine as a medical speciality has led to an analysis of palliative care as medicalized and colonized, leading to a readiness to resort to ever more medical interventions than was previously thought appropriate in hospice care (Biswas 1993).

The use of more active forms of treatment is both a source of tension, and also conceptual confusion among practitioners of palliative care. The tendency of palliative care to turn its attention 'upstream' from the terminal phase, to a much earlier point in the disease process, has been widely observed (Clark 2002). This coupled with the wider inclusiveness of diseases, other than cancer, has meant that forms of intervention are now used, which from a hospice perspective would have been judged as *extraordinary* and, hence, not justified. There is a magnitude of difference between what might be judged appropriate in the final days of life compared to what is justified at a point much earlier in the illness trajectory (Ellershaw and Ward 2003). Because the boundary around what is an appropriate or inappropriate treatment has become much less distinct, there has been a further corollary in terms of the need to clarify and justify the role of palliative interventions. Nevertheless, the emphasis of palliative care remains the control of symptoms and improving quality of life rather than curing the primary disease (WHO 2002).

The emphasis on comfort and the relief of suffering gives significant priority to the subjective states of the patient; suggesting that these ought to be paramount in determining the priorities of care. This emphasis is, in turn, reflected in the ethical underpinnings of practice, which is patient- and family-centred, premised upon a principle of respect for persons, but under an over arching conception of the good of palliative care, a philosophy succinctly summarised by Saunders (2005). It is this philosophy which I have argued is under pressure from secular liberal ethics.

An important way in which respect for persons is applied in palliative care practice is the priority given to the person's report of their suffering and to the expression of their wishes. Respecting the wishes of the person for how they wish to live their life to its close is not simply a matter of caving in to consumer autonomy, as Randall and Downie (2006) have argued. The distinctive palliative care axiology, which I argued in chapter 4 as being rooted in a communitarian approach, is one in which constraints on individual choice are justified against a background assumption that there is a better alternative to a good end-of-life. This contrasts with the liberal justification for constraining individual choice, which is based upon a mutual respect for freedom from interference.

The palliative care approach, as I see it, is willing to respect patient's wishes so long as such wishes do not conflict with the particular good, which palliative care sees itself as advancing. The justification for using palliative interventions is therefore not solely a matter of clinical evidence and 'symptomatology', as Kearney has warned (Kearney 1992: 41). Palliative care also involves a body of values, which include beliefs about better and worse ways to die, and the means to achieve or avoid these possible dying processes (Wanzer et al. 1989; Rousseau 1996). The issue of terminal sedation is therefore a challenge for palliative care at a number of levels; what is or is not appropriate to control in order to achieve a good death? This is not only a point about whether it is right to hasten death and within what constraints, but also concerns whether it is justified to control the experiences of the dying person, or in the case of deep sedation, curtail experience completely?

Traditional Christian ars moriendi required that the dying person be alert and aware of their death lest they give in to temptation at this final and crucial moment. While it is implausible that this Christian myth has any influence on clinical management in contemporary palliative care, there is certainly a plausible parallel in the secular discourse, which surrounds the practises of sedation. The idea that the level of the mental awareness of the patient is a critical factor when judging the appropriateness of an intervention is a plausible secular parallel. When Gillian Craig argues 'Having decided that sedation is needed, the doctor must try to find a drug regime that relieves distress but does not prevent the patient from verbal communication with friends and relatives' (1994: 140), she endorses a notion that the patient's awareness is a necessary constraint on how sedation ought to be used. The claim seems clearly nested within the values of palliative care that I have outlined in chapters 3 and 4. Personal growth and reconciliation does at least seem a possibility when the patient is able to continue communicating with the people they care about.

By contrast, when Troug *et al.* (1991) argue that, when a patient has refused continued ventilation and demanded its withdrawal then sedation should not be administered; it is not clear to what values they are appealing. Do they mean to imply that the patient's awareness of their suffering is a condition of having their end-of-life decisions respected? This seems to be rather a punitive approach to respecting patient's wishes with no opportunity for the act to contribute to the quality of the dying.

Perhaps the more plausible motive for the 'Troug' approach is rooted in one of the most often expressed concerns that in deeply sedating a patient there may be little to distinguish sedation from killing. If this is the case then taking this 'defensive medicine' approach surely cannot be justified at the cost of a much worse dying experience for the patient. With these preliminary thoughts in mind I turn now to defining a concept of palliative sedation and the ethical boundaries of its use.

The role and value of experiences: are some experiences not worth having?

In setting out some of the parameters of the good death in chapter 2, I explored the role that the manipulation and avoidance of certain kinds of experience might play. Sedation is one of the direct ways in which a person's conscious states can be manipulated. Sedation can be medically indicated when a person is anxious, agitated or pathologically restless. The purpose of sedation is to bring about a state of relaxation both physical and mental, to bring about sleep and to subdue awareness of unpleasant experiences (Randall and Downie 1999).

Sedation may be used to induce rest and a state of relaxation, but is also used as a means of diminishing or avoiding the awareness of unpleasant experiences, such as distressing medical examinations like endoscopies. Sedation is also sometimes used by people who are being intensively treated for cancer and I shall use this example as a less controversial way of exploring the role of sedation in deliberately altering a person's experiences. In using this particular example I am seeking to establish that deliberately aiming to alter the experiences of the patient is a legitimate goal in the use of sedation. Establishing this will be an important step in developing the case for PS.

Cancer treatments that combine drug and radiation therapies can be very arduous for the patient especially when they cause severe nausea and vomiting. Such episodes may last several days or longer, despite the use of modern antiemetic drugs. Patients who have such a severe reaction become exhausted and psychologically very low, and in such cases a regime of sedation may be indicated using drugs such as benzodiazepines normally used to treat acute anxiety states. Administered intravenously, they can have a strong sedative effect and, in most case, people will sleep or experience a somnolent state for long periods. Although some people may continue to vomit during this time, they usually benefit from an amnesia induced by the drug, resulting in a few 'lost' days during the worst of the nausea and vomiting.

In the absence of a request not to be sedated by the patient, it is difficult to see how such a loss can be of any significance; indeed, most people are likely to consider such a loss to be a positive benefit. This example rings true with hedonistic theory, one of the philosophical accounts of the good life considered in chapter 2. Hedonism is the view that the goodness of a life is contingent upon the quality of the experiences a person has during that life. From the hedonist point of view, a good life is one in which pleasurable experiences outweigh unpleasant ones. I have previously described some of the limitations of a hedonist theory of the good life, but there is no escaping from the fact that one's capacity for living a good life is severely restricted if every waking moment is overshadowed by an acutely unpleasant experience, unremitting pain, agitation, nausea and vomiting or breathlessness. As I have suggested, a person is no worse off, indeed, intuitively one would consider him or her better off for not having to undergo, or at least *remember* undergoing a prolonged period of severe nausea and vomiting. This is not to say that a person could not find some meaning in the experience, the demanding nature of some cancer treatment might be regarded by some as a personally beneficial experience, knowing that you have fought bravely against a killer disease. Some people are able to find strength in the fact that they have coped with a serious illness and are able to bring this strength to bear on other aspects of their life. The possible meaning that people may find in their experiences of coping with challenging situations is boundless. However, whatever the meaning this experience may have for a person, it is the meaning he or she alone finds in the experience that endows it with value. This is not to say that others cannot be inspired vicariously by the fortitude and courage of others; we can and are. However, this benefit is strictly parasitic upon the value with which the person whose experience it is imbues that experience. Individuals may find meaning in suffering, and the principle may be a sound one, but to claim that there is virtue in the suffering of a person if they find no meaning or value in the experience is a corruption of the virtue. If this were not the case then a powerful motive for relieving the suffering of others would be removed.

An important principle in the contemporary management of pain and other symptoms is that the person who says they have pain, should be believed and their own testimony should be the main reference point when adjusting their pain relief. This principle is crucial to understanding what constitutes good care of people who are suffering pain or other symptoms. In addition to the relief of symptoms, there are also other virtues at play in caring for a suffering person. These virtues are seldom described in any detail in the ethics literature perhaps because they fall within the general category of beneficence, the usual level of abstraction at which these matters are discussed. However, these goods are often described when giving an account of the value of palliative care. It is the point that, even in the face of suffering, good palliative care may contribute to rendering a challenging experience, if not meaningful, then more bearable. In her early writings about the hospice experience Saunders used the metaphor of the 'vigil', watching with the patient (Saunders 2003). Nathanson gave an account of this practice as one of integral goods of palliative care while giving evidence to the House of Lords Select Committee regarding the *Assisted Dying for the Terminally Ill Bill* (ADTI):

> Palliative care does a great deal more than pain control or symptom control: it also gives a great deal of psychological support: ... I remember well one patient saying to me very explicit: "What I want to know is that I will not be abandoned: there will not be a stage when people will say 'There is nothing more we can do for you'."
> (House of Lords 2005b: 33)

Sedating a patient even to a point at which they are deeply asleep or comatose does not necessarily mean that the patient has been abandoned. Even if this patient were to be deeply sedated, they would still be cared for with respect and dignity; with someone watching over the them, turning them, keeping them clean, going to the bedside, quietly and discreetly, to observe and so on. Attending to these aspects of good care renders the use of deep sedation in the palliative context consistent and compatible with the palliative care value of maintaining respect for the person until their death.

In this example, I have used an account of a person receiving intensive and potentially curative treatment. However, would our intuitions differ if the lost days were at the end-of-life, rather than at some earlier point? Although I have argued that it is the person whose life it is who gives meaning to their life, even out of their suffering, it is also plausible that this would occur in moments of reflection at a time after the period of suffering. This is, of course, not an opportunity the dying person has. No doubt some people will wish to experience their life to its end, perhaps because they wish to cling to life itself or because they have a particular religious belief about the end of life; however, there can be no obligation to experience one's life to its end and, in many cases, not doing so can be a positive benefit in the same way that avoiding the experience of nausea is a benefit.

However, other ethically challenging aspects of terminal sedation also make the practice controversial and I now turn to consider some of these.

What is in a word?

Tännsjö's definition of TS as: 'a procedure where through heavy sedation a terminally ill patient is put into a state of coma, where the intention of the doctor is that the patient should stay comatose until he or she is dead'. Tännsjö's position is that terminal sedation can be distinguished from euthanasia and, furthermore, is an ethical alternative to euthanasia in countries where the general ethos is against euthanasia. I believe that such a distinction *is* feasible and that sedation ought to be considered a valid option at the end of life. I do not agree that *terminal* sedation is an appropriate description of this intervention, and I believe that the distinction between sedation and euthanasia is much harder to sustain when other decisions, for example, to withhold hydration and nutrition are not considered as distinct decisions in their own right.

Tännsjö also identifies three positions with regard to terminal sedation:

- that it should never take place;
- that it should take place, but only as a last resort;
- that it should be considered a normal part of palliative care and that a doctor should be free to provide it at the terminally ill patient's request.

Like Tännsjö, I find the third position defensible, but would also consider the second position as the one most compatible with the palliative care approach to care at the end of life.

Materstvedt and Kaasa (2000) first described some of the ethical problems associated with TS, they also suggested that *palliative* sedation should be the routine and preferred substitution for TS. Others have been quick to follow. Broeckaert has argued that the use of sedation in the context of palliative care is a valid palliative intervention (2002a, 2002b). He further argues that referring to the use of *terminal* sedation is ambiguous, misleading as to the nature and purpose of sedation, and does not sufficiently distinguish the practice from forms of euthanasia. Broeckaert's positive account of *palliative* sedation covers some useful ground and helps to show how sedation is compatible with good palliative care. The arguments also suggest ways in which sedation in the palliative context can be distinguished from euthanasia. I therefore intend to follow these suggestions and use the term 'palliative sedation' as a substitute for TS.

Broeckaert argues using an approach generally used within the palliative literature, that the use of the term 'terminal' is unnecessarily negative in its connotation. This is a familiar point from within the palliative care community, which over the past 40 years has attempted to define itself both as a new health speciality and as a speciality that makes an active contribution to the care of those with progressive diseases. In chapter 3, I described the UK context and the deliberate decision to adopt the term 'palliative' care in place of terms such as 'hospice' or 'terminal' care so as to convey something positive about the care of people with incurable disease from their diagnosis through to their death (Woods *et al.* 2001). This positive account is reflected in the WHO definition of palliative care and is to be found reflected in the many national statements of palliative care philosophy adopted by the numerous countries that have made a commitment to palliative care.

In addition to its negative connotations TS is also ambiguous on several fronts, semantically and conceptually. For one thing, a common understanding of 'terminal' is that it is synonymous with the terminus or end, and in this case, death. Palliative care, however, is not solely concerned with the terminal stages of a disease, but sees itself as engaged across the spectrum of active disease, which in many cases may be years from death. If sedation is an appropriate intervention for symptom relief, then what should the use of sedation in the non-terminal phase of care be called, 'non-terminal sedation'? The point is that any prefix seems redundant unless it contributes something meaningful to the term to which it is attached. This, in turn, raises the question as to the justification of using the term 'terminal sedation' in any context. Broekaert suggests that one reason not to use this expression is because it implies, falsely, a more active causal role for the sedation itself, which is suggestive of some form of euthanasia, a highly undesirable implication from the palliative care perspective. For one thing, using a term for a practice that carries such implications may disadvantage those who may stand to benefit. Patients who most likely would benefit from sedation might refuse to consent for fear that this was a form of euthanasia. Broeckaert suggests that a term is needed for this practice, which is clear both about the criteria for use and the intention behind the intervention; hence, 'palliative sedation'.

At first glance, it is not clear that the term 'palliative' is an improvement on other candidate terms. However, without becoming distracted with the details of the history of this term, it is quite clear that a consensus has emerged regarding palliative forms of treatment within the broader context of palliative care. I have previously outlined the impetus for the development of modern palliative care in chapter 3, this aimed at effective symptom control and to improve the quality of life of dying for people with incurable disease. From an early stage, there was the intention to achieve a balance or therapeutic ratio between the burden of medical interventions against the severity of symptoms and improvements in quality of life. One of the elements of this therapeutic ratio was the dilemma of under-treatment versus the problems of iatrogenesis. At this stage in the 1950s and 1960s little was known about the phenomenon of pain and the ways in which it could be treated. Although morphine was readily available, its mechanism was not fully understood and many doctors had such fear of causing side-effects that, when morphine was used, it was used in inadequate ways. The side-effects that doctors were concerned about included causing addiction, but more serious was the fear of causing premature death, because morphine may cause a fatal depression of the patient's breathing if the dosage is not closely related to the severity of their symptoms. However, on this latter point a different approach was adopted by some doctors who argued that, when there was no other way of relieving a patient's suffering, then side-effects, even fatal ones, are justified. It is here that the familiar justification for such practises, touched on by Tännsjö, comes into play. The argument is that treating a patient in such a way that the treatment shortens his or her life can be distinguished from murder or mercy killing because of the intention of the doctor to treat, rather than kill, and because the treatment used has more than one effect. This enables the doctor to *intend* the beneficial effect and *foresee,* but not intend the negative effect. This very point was made by Lord Devlin in a now famous English legal case, R v Adams [1957] where he commented:

> If the first purpose of medicine, the restoration of health, can no longer be achieved, there is still much for the doctor to do, and he is entitled to do all that is proper and necessary to relieve pain and suffering even if the measures he takes might incidentally shorten life.
> (*R v Bodkin Adams* [1957] CLR 365 (CCC) Devlin J)

This introduction into English law of the doctrine of double effect (DDE) has been the cause of extensive debate, much of which is relevant to the issue of terminal sedation. It is necessary therefore to spend some time on this distinction, but for the moment I shall do so in relation to the treatment of pain. I, like Tännsjö, believe that there is a plausible defence of the DDE and I shall argue for this in the context of palliative care.

One of the central criticisms of the DDE is made by those who see the consequences of an act as the determinant of the moral character of the act. Hence, when two acts lead to equivalent outcomes they are therefore *morally* equivalent acts. This is the point made by Kuhse and others when they say that bringing about a person's death by an act, which foresees, but does not intend their death as a consequence, is morally equivalent to directly and intentionally bringing about their death. I shall say nothing further on this point here other than to state that both intentions and consequences in my view are relevant to the moral nature of an act.

Here, I shall discuss a second criticism of the DDE, which concentrates on the role ascribed by its supporters to intention. Critics of the DDE argue on two grounds, first is that it is difficult, if not impossible to distinguish intending from merely foreseeing an effect. Second, because intentions are subjective states there is the problem of verifying just what the intention of the actor was in a given situation.

While it may be difficult and sometimes impossible to distinguish intending from foreseeing, it is surely not the case that it is always *impossible* to judge another's intentions. If it were so, it would be impossible to convict in the criminal courts, which relies on a verdict beyond all reasonable doubt. To judge what another intended relies not only upon first person testimony, an insight, if the person is truthful, into the *subjective* conditions of their intention, but also on the *objective* conditions, the facts of the matter, what they did and how they acted. Of course, this is not to say that this is an infallible approach; indeed, there are uses of the DDE in which the minimal or sufficient conditions for rendering an act 'innocent' are met, but in such a way as to obscure the real intentions at play. I refer to this as the 'Cynical Doctrine of Double Effect'. The legal case *R v Adams* [1957] is perhaps one such example where the doctor (Adams) was acquitted of deliberately ending the lives of his patients by increasing the dosage of opiates administered to them, in circumstances in which he stood to inherit money from his patients. Adams was acquitted because his actions met certain sufficient conditions, his patients were terminally ill and he used an appropriate drug, an opiate, to relieve their suffering.

In a similar case, but one lacking the implications of personal gain, *R v Moor* [1999], Dr Moor was accused of murdering a patient because he admitted to using lethal doses of morphine on this terminally ill man. Dr Moore was also acquitted, despite his avowed sympathies with euthanasia, because he had used an appropriate drug to treat the suffering of his terminally ill patient. The Court came to a different conclusion in the case of *R. v Cox* [1992] in which a Dr Cox was convicted of attempted murder when his patient Lillian Boyes died following an injection of potassium chloride. Cox was convicted because his chosen means, potassium chloride, has no analgesic effect and had no therapeutic uses in the circumstances, thereby falling short of one of the sufficient conditions for a 'tolerated' act, since he could not claim that potassium chloride had a double effect. Had Dr Cox killed Lillian Boyes with an opiate then it is highly unlikely that his action would have resulted in a conviction. In reporting these cases, I make no comment on the detail or the debated ethical status of each, I merely use them to indicate that an action can be seen to meet the conditions of the DDE, placing the act in the class of tolerated interventions, even when there are reasons to suspect they are acts of a different moral kind. A more relevant example of the cynical version of the DDE is the once familiar and, I believe, not entirely eradicated practice of placing a dying person on a morphine infusion. The use of the infusion is accompanied by a prescription for an escalating dose of morphine to be continued until they are dead. I believe that some acts of this kind have cynically employed the DDE to disguise actions that fall into the upper left 'forbidden' quadrant of

Tännsjö's matrix; and the most troubling of these are cases in which no reference is made to the patient's wishes. On these grounds I am in agreement with those who argue that the DDE allows euthanasia by subterfuge.

However, one way in which the cynical uses of the DDE can be exposed is to focus more closely on the objective conditions of the DDE and, hence, to focus more closely on the objective aspects of an action as a 'good enough' indicator of the actor's intention. This, in turn, raises questions about the standards of care and what constitutes an appropriate intervention. Research into palliative care, especially research that has attempted to delineate and clarify palliative interventions, is very relevant here. Earlier, I referred to the ignorance that existed around pain and its effective treatment, particularly by the use of opiates, which led to either ineffective treatment or premature death. However, since that time the groundbreaking work of, among others, Robert Twycross (1990) into the pharmacokinetics and clinical uses of opiates has standardized the use of opiates for pain and other symptom relief.

The principles of appropriate palliative treatment lie in the twin concepts of adequacy and proportionality. Hence, an intervention is justified if the treatment is adequate for the task and is proportionate in its effect to the symptoms the patient is experiencing. Twycross and Lack (1993) give many practical examples of the principles of managing a patient's pain with morphine. Having established that a patient's pain is, in fact, responsive to opiates then the aim is to stabilize the patient on a regime that keeps them comfortable with the minimum of side-effects. If a patient experiences pain, while taking morphine then they give the following advice: 'The aim is to increase the dose progressively until the patient's pain is relieved (dose titration). The patient (sic) should be advised to increase the dose by 50 per cent if the first dose is not more effective than the previous medication ...' (1993: 11). Through this method, it is possible to manage a person, pain free and conscious on a dosage of morphine, which would likely be fatal to a person naïve to the drug, indicating that even a large dosage of morphine can be proportionate. This stands in clear contrast to the scenario I described earlier where patients are placed on an escalating dosage of morphine or the legal cases in which patient's were arguably administered a disproportionate dose of opiate, that is, without reference to the patient's levels of comfort or tolerance of the drug. It is therefore possible to obtain objective evidence of the intention behind an intervention, which may expose important differences between ostensibly similar acts. In Law, this possibility has informed the legal standard in negligence, and in the English courts it is known as the 'Bolam Standard', which states that: 'A doctor is not guilty of negligence if he has acted in accordance with a practice accepted as proper by a responsible body of medical men skilled in that particular art' (*Bolam v Friern Hospital Management Committee* [1957] 2

All ER 118). The approach I suggest is described by Huxtable as the '*Bolam*-ization of *Adams*' (2004: 67), and as he discusses, this move still leaves the fundamental law on murder unchanged, resulting in the undesirable conclusion that some practitioners may be seen as murderers, albeit 'justified' murderers. There is, therefore, probably no substitute for a fundamental review of the law on murder as it applies to these contexts.

The approach, I suggest, also leaves open the possibility that there may be differences of opinion between different bodies, but in the context of palliative care a great deal of effort has been made to identify and clarify the principles and standards of practice. While this does not render disagreement impossible, it shows that it is possible to give evidence of demonstrable consensus, which in the context of pain control makes it possible to expose the cynical exploitation of the DDE.

I have spent some time discussing the principles of palliative care in the context of pain relief because I now wish to go on to show how these principles can be applied to sedation in palliative care. There is, however, an important caveat since there is nothing like as strong a consensus on what constitutes the 'gold standard' of treatment with regard to sedation, in the way that morphine is to pain. However, I believe that the principles of palliative care are robust enough to establish some of the parameters.

There is no doubt that sedation is appropriate in the palliative care context, whether this is to aid in bringing sleep, relieve anxiety or to augment the effects of analgesics. However, such uses of sedation fall within the range of normal clinical indications, but *palliative* sedation is employed in circumstances where a reduction in consciousness is the only means of relieving a person's suffering because their symptoms are refractory to the standard treatment. This is consistent with the goals of palliative care, which aims at the patient's comfort, rather than cure.

Having discussed the principles of palliative care in relation to pain management it should now begin to be clear why Materstvedt and Kaasa's (2000) suggestion that the use of sedation in the palliative care context should be referred to as *palliative* sedation. This is not because the term is specific to all circumstances, but rather because it implies specific criteria that must be met in order to justify its use, the key principles of adequacy and proportionality.

Broeckaert offers the following definition: Palliative sedation is:

> ... the intentional administration of sedatives in such dosages and combinations as required to reduce the terminal patient's consciousness as much as needed to adequately control one or more refractory symptoms.
>
> (Broeckaert 2000)

Broeckaert's definition leaves open the possibility that the sedation used might be light or heavy, constant, periodic or temporary, and hence there is scope for individualizing and reviewing the effectiveness of the use of sedation in particular cases. Any person who is suffering can be relieved of their suffering by being rendered deeply and permanently unconscious. The difficulty I have with Tännsjö's use and definition of terminal sedation, as set out above, is that it describes only the most extreme end of the spectrum of palliative sedation, and does not consider the issue of withholding hydration and nutrition as distinct decisions. Adopting Tännsjö's approach in all cases will not be sensitive to the spectrum of appropriate uses of sedation nor to the range of desires individuals may have with regard to how they live out their last days.

Whether an intervention is adequate and proportionate can be judged by attending to a number of issues:

• How was the treatment instigated?
• Are symptoms refractory to conventional treatment?
• Who instigated the decision to sedate?
• If the patient is competent was consent obtained?
• Was a second opinion sought?

There are many symptoms, which may become refractory, including pain, agitation and dyspnea, for which sedation may be considered an appropriate palliative intervention. I do not intend to discuss such symptoms here, however, I do wish to raise the question of whether psychological or *existential* suffering ought to be regarded as a symptom for which sedation is indicated (Chernoy 1998). It should be clear from the preceding discussion that I believe this to be the case in the context of terminal illness. It is not difficult to imagine the circumstances in which a person may come to experience the mere awareness of their continued existence as a cause of suffering. As with any other symptom the person's 'self report' must be taken at face value and responded to. Nor is it difficult to envisage that such suffering may also be refractory to a range of interventions of a pharmacological, psychological and even spiritual kind. It is in such circumstances that the use of deep and prolonged sedation, of the kind envisaged in Tännsjö's definition of TS, seems appropriate. Of course, such interventions are not without precedent within the palliative care context and, as such, are compatible with a concept of good palliative care. As I have reported, to sedate a person even to the point of unconsciousness could be challenged ethically if this amounted to abandoning the person. However, as I have argued, the practice within palliative care is to care for the person with respect and gentleness in just the same way that a dying person unconscious through the disease process would be cared for.

It might be objected that responding in such a way to existential suffering is characteristic only of some aspects of western medicine and the extremes to which it resorts out of obsessive devotion to patient autonomy. However, this objection cannot be sustained. Such practises are also acceptable to cultures normally seen as antithetical to the autonomy-centric Northern European and Anglo-American traditions. Nunez-Olarte and Gracia (2001) comment on Spain, a country with a relatively mature palliative care service, but culturally Southern European and Catholic. They cite Spain's rejection of euthanasia, but acceptance of:

> pain relief to the point of sedation, even in cases where death might be accelerated. Within the Catholic tradition, the Thomistic principle of double effect, broadly developed by the Spanish 'School of Salamanca' in the sixteenth century is commonly used by Spanish physicians to support the use of analgesics and sedatives.
>
> (Nunez-Olarte and Gracia 2001: 57)

The implication for terminal care is the phenomenon of 'Spanish Death', marked by a readiness to respond to psychological or spiritual suffering with sedation, which '... implies that unconsciousness, either disease- or drug-induced, is generally perceived as the 'best way out', especially when patients are aware of their prognosis, regardless of whether life is shortened by the use of these drugs' (2001: 58).

My conclusion, therefore, is that sedation, even deep sedation, where it is adequate and proportionate, is an appropriate palliative intervention and is consistent with the ethics and values of palliative care. Sedation can be initiated in response to refractory physical symptoms, where the depth and duration of the sedation is proportionate to the symptoms. Sedation can be doctor instigated with the consent of a competent patient or in the patient's best interests where the patient lacks capacity. Sedation may also be instigated at the patient's request for reasons of psychological or existential suffering, although the deep continuous sedation of a person who is not imminently dying might only be acceptable if there were no alternative measures which the patient could be persuaded to try. The greatest ethical challenge arises in the case of a terminally ill person who requests deep sedation because of their existential suffering, and who has been eating and drinking normally and, although terminally ill, is relatively physically stable. This scenario is perhaps closest to the extreme case of terminal sedation set out by Tännsjö.

This is challenging because a person who is terminally ill is not necessarily a person who is imminently dying. So what is compatible with palliative care of a person who is terminally ill, but *not* imminently dying? Assuming also that the person is conscious and competent, then it is difficult to imagine a set of circumstances in which an ethically- or legally-justified decision could be made to feed and hydrate a competent patient who has refused.

On the matter of the patient's request for deep sedation, then much will hinge upon whether existential suffering is accepted as a symptom and whether this symptom is refractory to conventional treatment. Even among

those who are not sceptical with regard to the validity of existential suffering, it would be difficult to find a consensus as to what constituted the
standard treatment against which the symptoms can be said to be refractory: anxiolytics, psychotherapy or spiritual counselling? However, on the
principle that it is the person him or herself who is the authority as to their
own suffering, then their own report should be believed and acted upon.
Therefore, a person who is terminally ill, but who is not imminently dying,
yet complains of existential suffering must be in a position to receive
appropriate treatment, that is adequate treatment which is proportionate to
their needs; and therefore treatment with deep sedation as a last resort must
remain an option. If sedation is combined with a competent refusal of
artificial hydration and nutrition — then this seems to present a potential
scenario in which terminal sedation of the kind described by Tännsjö may
be instigated in a palliative care setting. Palliative care is not committed to
the view that dying people are under an obligation to experience their own
dying process nor is it conceivable that imposing such awareness on a dying
person, by refusing their request for sedation, could be justified.

By now, it should be clear that much of what I have said in examining the
question of terminal sedation in palliative care has areas of agreement, but
some significant disagreement with Tännsjö's position outlined at the start
of this chapter. Significantly, I have argued for a more cautious approach to
the definition. At best Tännsjö's definition describes one extreme end of the
spectrum of the justified use of sedation in terminally ill patients. For this
reason, I agree with Materstvedt and Kaasa (2000), Broeckaert (2000) and
with other commentators that the term 'palliative sedation' is a more
appropriate one. Where I disagree with Tännsjö's position is over his
inclusion of decisions regarding hydration and nutrition as part of the same
clinical decision to utilize sedation; this as far as possible should be
regarded as a related, but distinct decision. I have by no means exhausted
all of the circumstances in which decisions to combine sedation with
treatment withdrawal may be legitimate. Consistent with the account I
support one could envisage the use of deep sedation combined with the use
of artificial hydration, but withholding other forms of treatment such as
antibiotics and ventilation.

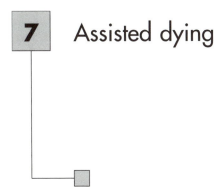

7 | Assisted dying

Introduction

In this chapter I will discuss assisted dying and a range of measures to hasten death from euthanasia to assisted suicide. In other words, this chapter is about killing. I begin with this statement because I have given careful thought to the question of the most appropriate form of words to use to refer to these acts. I wish to acknowledge from the start that all measures to hasten death are forms of killing, but nevertheless my preferred term will be 'assisted dying'. To use this expression is, I suppose, to use a euphemism that will probably not sit well with those who, on the one hand, are opposed to any form of deliberate killing and, on the other hand, who believe some killing is acceptable but we should be honest about it. Both camps might turn with contempt and argue that no form of sophistry can disguise the fact that ending a life *is* killing and, in the first camp, killing is wrong, and in the second camp, killing is sometimes right. I wish to use the term 'assisted dying' because I wish to include in this category not only the most obvious candidates of euthanasia and assisted suicide, but also the other means of assisting death. In the category of 'other means' I also include symptom control and sedation that assist the dying process by engineering the parameters of the good death without interfering with, what for some remains, a 'natural death'. In extending this category, I aim to argue for a concept of 'appropriate' killing, a concept that is, in my view, compatible with the palliative care values, although I believe that the palliative care community is a long way from being able to acknowledge this possibility.

Even among those who take the strongest stance against killing, it is rare to find individuals who are absolute in this regard (Oderberg 2000a, b). Those who are broadly opposed to killing usually accommodate their position to allow killing of certain kinds (Geddes 1973). Oderberg, who defends a version of what he calls 'traditional morality', argues for the sanctity of *innocent* life, but finds this position consistent with killing in self-defence, killing in the context of a just war, capital punishment and the ending even of innocent life where this is the foreseen, but unintended consequence of a 'good' act. The practical difficulty with such absolute positions is, as I argued in chapter 1, that they grate against ordinary moral intuitions when it comes to accounting for right action in complex moral contexts. Khuse (2002) comments on Geddes' (1973) defence of certain obstetric practises, which seem to entail killing the innocent, as: 'an ingenious exercise in sophistry' (2002: 271).

These brief points suggest that, even among those who claim to support the sanctity-of-life doctrine, it is possible to distinguish between different forms of killing and more importantly between the *moral* character of these acts. My first task, in this chapter, is to map out some of these important distinctions. My second and main task will be to develop the concept of appropriate killing, and to argue that this form of assisted dying is compatible with palliative care.

Whatever one's position on these matters, I believe that we should all find killing, the deliberate ending of life, morally problematic and take pause to reflect upon the reasons that might justify or prohibit such actions. One of the crucial questions to be addressed here is whether we can draw moral distinctions between superficially similar acts? I believe we can, and that attempting to make such distinctions is both an indication and a requirement of moral progress.

In this chapter, the focus of my discussion will be quite broad, but will move to give special consideration to palliative care, but where my argument requires it I will discuss other examples including some outside of the health context.

Given the focus of my discussion, it seems even more appropriate to reject talk of killing and to talk of assisted dying. When we talk of someone who dies after the withdrawal of artificial nutrition and hydration, or ventilation then it is morally misleading to ask 'was he killed?' To answer either 'yes' or 'no' to this question is to mislead in distinct, but equally problematic ways. To answer 'yes' implies that there must be a killer or killers, a harsh and I would argue an invalid implication in circumstances such as those of the person who is permanently unconscious. To answer 'no' in circumstances where a person is ventilator dependent, but otherwise stable, that is, not dying in any ordinary sense of the term. Then 'no' seems to imply an implausible lack of a causal connection between such withdrawals and the death of the individual (Stauch 2002).

There is good reason, then, to be cautious about the terms used in such a reflection since talk of killing is inevitably emotive, indeed disturbing, the word is associated with killers, murderous criminals who take life with malicious intent and not usually with any form of care. The concept of killing and the concept of care are taken by many as mutually exclusive concepts, but without scratching the surface of such concepts we cannot be certain of their soundness in our moral deliberations. Attention to the form of words used is therefore necessary to the purposes of this chapter because I wish to explore the possibility of drawing moral distinctions between the different forms of ending life and so would seek to avoid obscuring such distinctions by masking them with morally loaded terms such as 'killing'. However, relevant to this task are the legal frameworks within which such terms also derive their meaning. In English law there have been frequent calls to recognize a category of 'mercy killing' within the law on homicide. Although, the very juxtaposition of those words is problematic, attempting to categorise an act that appears morally contradictory. A culpable killing, a murder that is also merciful? Although the Criminal Law Revision Committee has rejected this opinion, the way in which the law has dealt with a number of ostensibly mercy killings is itself telling. Acts of so-called mercy killing have resulted in convictions for murder, manslaughter and what might be viewed as convictions of an ambiguous kind in which the sanctions imposed by the court have been so minimal or non-existent even, so as to imply that the acts are of a different moral kind to plain murder (*R. v Cox* [1992]). The fact of such discrimination implies that there are grounds on which such distinctions are made. Given that the law is only a guide to what is lawful and not necessarily what is ethical, the legal framework may mark the point of departure from our moral understanding and evaluation of these issues. Indeed, many of the end-of-life problems encountered in the English Courts in recent years have been complicated by a too narrow legal definition of murder or assisted suicide, requiring the Courts to engage in verbal gymnastics in order to defend certain medical practises (*Airedale NHS Trust v Bland* [1993], Re: B (Adult refusal of Medical treatment) [2002], Huxtable 2004).

Assisted dying: definition of terms

The usual place to start with any discussion of euthanasia is with a definition of terms and the now standard taxonomy of the various forms of euthanasia. The literal meaning of the term euthanasia: a good or happy death, has been rendered redundant by the contemporary meaning of intentionally bringing about the death of an individual. Perhaps the most common, but not necessarily the least controversial usage of the term is within veterinary medicine, where euthanasia refers to the ending of an animal's life by direct and painless means. The same definition has been applied to the human context but with the attention to the following further distinctions:

Figure 7.1   Taxonomy of euthanasia

Active euthanasia	Passive euthanasia
Voluntary	Voluntary
Non-voluntary	Non-voluntary
Involuntary	Involuntary

Taxonomy of euthanasia

These further distinctions are necessary in the human context, but not the veterinary, since notions of consent or voluntariness are not relevant in the non-human animal context (see Figure 7.1). By contrast, notions of mercy and compassion seem straightforwardly applicable to the animal context, whereas in the human context they are somewhat double-edged for the contrary reason. One of the grounds of what is permissible in the human context is defined in terms of *a* if not *the* most fundamental concept; consent or voluntariness.

I am not suggesting that consent is a sufficient condition of the morally permissible, but rather that it is, at least in circumstances where a person is capable of consenting. 'Mercy' and 'compassion' are, by contrast, motives quite independent of consent. Mercy and compassion may be motivated by genuine concerns for the welfare of a suffering patient, but this does not justify overriding the person's will. We have previously encountered the liberal justification for respect for autonomy, which puts the point in the most robust of terms; where a person is conscious and competent and does not wish their life to end, then no welfare concern can justify overriding their will and most people will agree that this is the principal wrong of murder.

With the few notable exceptions, including the Netherlands and Belgium, most jurisdictions follow that of the UK in regarding all of the categories in the first column as unlawful and also, but less emphatically, as unethical. Whereas the categories represented in the second column are regarded as both lawful and ethical. Indeed, the second column is now generally regarded as controversial if presented in a context in which the categories are seen to imply any kind of euthanasia at all, although Doyal's arguments in favour of non-voluntary active euthanasia give a number of compelling reasons as to why this should be regarded as a permissible form of euthanasia (Doyal 2006). Actions that might result in deaths, classified in this column, include the withholding or withdrawing of life-sustaining treatment, where such treatment is regarded as futile and the cause of death will inevitably be due to the underlying condition. This class of death would also include competent refusals of life-sustaining treatment.

The distinction between the first and second columns reflects the position endorsed by the European Association for Palliative Care (EAPC) whose ethics task force issued a position statement on euthanasia and physician assisted suicide (Materstvedt *et al.* 2003). Within this statement, the category that I have identified within the table as passive involuntary euthanasia is dismissed. The EAPC task force deny that such a category is even conceptually possible, because in their view, by definition, all forms of euthanasia are active. Passive euthanasia is therefore not *euthanasia*, but is a 'contradiction in terms' (Materstvedt *et al.* 2003: 98). The thought that life-sustaining treatment may be withheld or withdrawn from a competent patient, without their consent and against their will, does of course sound barbaric. Yet this was the very issue that was brought to the English Courts by Oliver Burke, a man with a degenerative neurological condition, who believed he may find himself in exactly this position (Evans 2004). This case demonstrates in the clearest possible terms that the possibility of *involuntary* passive euthanasia is perceived as a real issue by individuals who feel vulnerable to such a practice. Oliver Burke specifically challenged the General Medical Council's (GMC) guidelines for withholding and withdrawing life-prolonging treatments (GMC 2002). Mr Burke's concern was that when the time came that he was no longer able to eat or drink naturally, he would wish to be fed artificially, but the GMC (2002) suggest that such support may be denied or withdrawn from him by his doctors. Mr Burke took his case to the Courts because he wished to be fed and provided with hydration until his death by natural causes. (*R (Burke) v – The General Medical Council* [2003]). Mr Burke's circumstances do, therefore, seem to present a potential case of involuntary and passive euthanasia, if one accepts, as Mr Burke believed, that his death may be caused by not receiving ANH.

Mr Burke's case eventually went to the Court of Appeal where it was overturned. The GMC guidelines, which, although criticized, were vindicated by the Court of Appeal, thus supporting the opinion that treatment may be withdrawn or withheld, where medical judgement regards such treatment as futile, irrespective of whether the patient has requested that the treatment continue or be instigated. Although this decision may seem to vindicate the EAPC's position it does nothing to ameliorate the concerns expressed by Mr Burke, which were taken so seriously by the judge at first instance. In summing up, the judge, J Munby, commented upon a number of aspects of Mr Burke's case that, in his opinion, were in breach of Human Rights legislation, in particular, he stated that, in principle, it is for a competent patient, and not his or her doctor, to decide what treatment should or should not be given 'in order to achieve what the patient believes conduces to his dignity and in order to avoid what the patient would find distressing'. Mr Burke's concerns present a challenge to which the palliative care community, indeed the whole of medicine, must respond and not merely by dismissing this as a contradictory moral category. The 'issues' in this and similar cases may justifiably be seen as issues of communication and trust, rather than issues of killing and letting die; but for the patient, and their concerned family, these may be distinctions that are hard to pull apart.

Before moving on, there are two points I wish to make from this digression into the EAPC position. The first is that, as with all position statements, there is a tendency to stipulate definitions in such a way that the complexity and ambiguity of certain moral problems are glossed over. The stipulation that all euthanasia is active, and that all non- or involuntary killings are murder, does not admit to the complexity that is typical of cases like that of Mr Burke. However, I do accept that it is necessary to posit a position in order that these issues be debated and for such debate to inform the formulation of a framework for practice. Such formulations also offer a focus for future revision. The second point is that the EAPC position, in so far as this reflects the opinions of the palliative care community, reveals a number of implicit ethical values including the acceptance that there are justified constraints on how far others are required to comply with an individual's autonomous wishes. This, as I have argued, is consistent with a communitarian interpretation of palliative care values and I shall be returning to this point later in my discussion.

Returning now to the classification of euthanasia in Figure 7.1, the category that is arguably least morally problematic, in the sense that it presents least room for debate, because it is closest to the kind of action universally condemned, is that of involuntary active euthanasia. This category does represent cases of straightforward murder and is therefore wrong for all the reasons that murder is condemned. However, even within the category of involuntary killing it is possible, and indeed right, to draw some important distinctions. Involuntary killing with 'malice aforethought' seems to occupy a different moral category from involuntary killing with 'benevolence aforethought'. This is uncomfortable territory for those who prefer to see a good patch of clear blue water between moral categories, but we should not rely upon moral discomfort alone as a guide to what is the right thing to do. I am not, of course, suggesting that involuntary mercy killing is something that we should accept routinely as the right thing to do. I do, however, wish to suggest that some such cases may be distinguished from what is a case of straightforward murder and the grounds of such distinctions are worthy of consideration.

Conspicuous by their absence from this taxonomy are the various classifications of suicide. Suicide could be redefined in such a way as to fit the above schema as: 'self-euthanasia' and 'assisted euthanasia' with a further distinction between the competent suicide and the competence-compromised suicide. The former might be characterized by the person with a terminal illness who chooses the time and means of their death, the latter a person whose suicidal urge is the result of a mental illness; itself amenable to treatment. Individuals in the latter group might include those who having failed in their suicide attempt, go on to receive appropriate treatment, recognize their suicidal behaviour as alien to their own interests and so go on to live their life without attempting suicide again (Glover 1984).

The example I give of a justified suicide, as a person with a terminal illness, could well be regarded as controversial by many; why choose terminal illness as an obvious justification? A point frequently made from the disability perspective is that able-bodied people rarely question the rationality of disabled people desiring suicide or seeking euthanasia (Bassnet 2002). Disability and terminal illness are, of course, not equivalent, as many disabled people are not terminally ill. However, the criticism cited is still well made since some might believe that my example implies that merely having a terminal illness suggests that a person would be better off dead. This is not the implication I wish to make, although I believe that having a terminal illness is a sufficient reason as to why someone may contemplate suicide. Contemplating suicide in the face of a terminal illness, as with any contemplation of suicide, may be more or less rational. As with irrational suicide generally; we ought to prevent them. Indeed, this is exactly the sort of suicidal contemplation that palliative care services may be uniquely placed to respond to, by treating depression, palliating symptoms, and by providing practical help and a supportive and nurturing environment. However, I believe that for the reasons explored in chapter 2, some suicides should not be prevented. As I have argued, suicide might provide the means of engineering some of the parameters of the good death, including the manner and timing of death.

Acknowledging this aspect of suicide is part of the basis of our moral anxiety about suicide. Our moral concern is not with suicides, which arise from pathological or other compelling influence, since there seems to be a *prima facie* reason for intervening and preventing such; it is rather with the 'rational' suicide. Those who support the right to bring one's life to an end through suicide or to have assistance in doing so, argue that there is a *right* to suicide; and when this cannot be achieved by one's own hand, this right leads to a claim of a right to assistance. This is a point that has been made very forcefully in a number of well publicized cases in the UK such as Diane Pretty, Reginald Crew and Ms B (Boyd 2002).

In chapter 2, I explored the plausibility of deliberately 'squaring off' as a means of engineering a good death; I have also considered the liberal arguments for autonomy and self-determination, both of which are relevant to this debate. The general move away from the criminalization of suicide, it is argued, is a mark of moral progress and a reflection of society's recognition of this right. However, whether the decriminalization of suicide amounts to the establishment of a right to suicide was a point hotly disputed in the case of Diane Pretty (Boyd 2002), a woman with multiple sclerosis who appealed to the House of Lords to allow her claimed right to assisted suicide. Diane Pretty's appeal was rejected and, as Lord Bingham's ruling argues, the decriminalizing of suicide does not establish such a right. The decriminalization of suicide in the UK took place with the amendment to The Suicide Act (1961), but rather than establishing a legal right, is regarded, rather as a response to the practical impossibility of enforcing such a law and also for the humane recognition that a person who fails in suicide usually deserves compassion and not prosecution.

As far as the legal position in England is concerned, changes in the legal status of suicide do not represent a right to commit suicide since assisting a suicide is, under the Act, punishable by a long prison sentence. Although the ambiguous and arbitrary application of the law, as *Dignity in Dying* (2006) points out, gives mixed messages. I shall come to the suggestions for further changes in English law later in this chapter. For now, the question is whether there are circumstances in which taking one's own life is justified — and both the denial and justification of this claim are problematic. The moral position implied by most jurisdictions, suggests that there are limits to individual freedom and that such constraints are a necessary condition of social living and, therefore, of human life; but these limits are not set in stone, they can and need to be challenged in the face of social change. This is the position explored in chapter 4, and the position I have argued as most compatible with the communitarian approach to palliative care values. However, I have already begun to make the case for the possibility of a rational and justified suicide in the case of a terminally ill person. One important complexity arises when that person lacks the ability to carry out the act.

In most contexts, it is accepted that while a person may commit suicide, it is wrong for another to assist them and, hence, justified to restrict autonomy by law and by social sanction. Such constraints on individual autonomy are not incompatible with the fundamental principle of law that the individual has an inviolable right to self-determination; since this is regarded as limiting what others may legitimately do to you and not what you may *require* others to do to you. However, as the cases of Oliver Burke and Ms B, albeit in different senses, have shown there is a growing willingness to challenge this position in the medical context. It is generally thought that to endorse a more robust form of self-determination, which might give substance to one's claim on others, would be to court anarchy, to allow self-determination to run amok. I will now consider this claim in the context of other positions on bringing life to an end.

Self-determination run amok

Daniel Callahan (1992) coined this memorable expression in a paper in which he identified the euthanasia debate as marking a profound turning point in Western thought. Callahan argued that accepting euthanasia would have implications for the legitimate conditions under which one person may kill another, the meaning and limits of self-determination, and our understanding of the goals of medicine. Callahan is candid that such a turn would be a turn for the worse.

Although there is an extensive literature arguing both for and against euthanasia and assisted dying, I have chosen Callahan's paper because it combines, in a short paper, many of the standard ethical arguments with a number of powerful intuitions. Callahan begins his argument with an implicit appeal to the intuition that, unreflectively, every decent-minded individual might feel compelled to endorse, namely the sanctity of life, or as we might pragmatically comprehend it, the *wrongness* of killing. Here, Callahan is clearly in good company, a view not only in keeping with what many people would regard as *the* most fundamental moral principle, but a principle also endorsed by every major world religion, state and legislature. Even among disparate moral thinkers there is consensus on the immorality of killing if not a consensus on the grounds for the wrongness of killing.

Callahan's argument therefore sweeps us along with the raw intuition that killing is wrong and that euthanasia as a form of killing is therefore to be condemned. Allowing euthanasia, Callahan argues, would mark a *volte-face* in our advancing civilization that has up to now sought ever more effective ways to *restrict* killing, rather than facilitate it. Let us first consider the details of Callahan's arguments before reflecting on their substance.

Callahan's moral concern is raised by the argument in favour of active voluntary euthanasia (AVE) because he believes it signifies an important moral turning point in Western thinking. He has three concerns. The first concerns the grounds on which one person may kill another. AVE would sanction 'consenting adult killing', adding a new category of killing to a society that already over-indulges in such acts. The second concerns our understanding of the right to self-determination. In Callahan's view the rights of the wider community with which an individual's rights must be compatible delimit the individual's right to self-determination. Allowing AVE is tantamount to saying that individuals take priority over the wider community. Callahan's third concern is that allowing AVE would bend the purposes of medicine to the purposes of individuals, rather than allowing medicine to pursue its proper role of promoting and pursuing health. For Callahan these turning points are turns in the wrong direction. Callahan is not alone in arguing this position, the arguments for and against euthanasia, for and against killing have been made many times, and although this chapter covers some of this same well trodden territory I hope eventually to offer a new perspective on palliative care in this context.

I want to take up two points made by Callahan before moving on. The first is to examine the moral intuition that killing is wrong and here I wish to deny that the generally shared intuition that killing is wrong equates to a shared agreement on the sanctity of life. The second is to consider his account of the limits of personal autonomy because this echoes some of my own arguments about autonomy and respect for persons in palliative care. First, then, the wrongness of killing and, as I have said, most people would accept the raw intuition that killing is wrong. However, the intuition is less clear once we begin to unpack what is actually meant by 'killing', as I have already begun to set out earlier in this chapter.

Suicide is a useful place to begin this analysis because, as Callahan, admits suicide may at least form the basis of an argument for a right to end one's life; a right to kill if only one's self. Although Callahan suggests that if suicide is regarded as a solitary act, it therefore falls within the realms of self-determination and is unlike AVE, which of necessity requires the involvement of another. This, of course, is to take a very simplified view of suicide, which is as much a social phenomenon as it is a solitary act; however, this is to digress.

The moral stumbling block for Callahan is therefore the move from my right to end my life to the right of another to act as my killer. Callahan goes on: 'The idea that we can waive our right to life, and then give to another the power to take that life, requires a justification yet to be provided by anyone' (1992: 52).

This seems a particularly strong claim without further justification. Callahan might well be calling upon a fundamental tenet of the American Constitution to protect 'life and Liberty', which itself harkens to a much older tradition of which the Constitution is arguably a manifestation, what Oderberg calls 'traditional morality' (2000b: viii). A cornerstone of traditional morality is the doctrine of the sanctity of life. Orderberg states this simply as:

> *Doctrine of the Sanctity of Life (DSL)*: It is always and everywhere a grave moral wrong intentionally to take the life of an *innocent* human being. (2000a: 147 emphasis added)

However, Callahan's claim, and for that matter Oderberg's, and any other defender of the traditional version of this doctrine, seems to be far too strong. It is not possible to simply 'read off' from the doctrine as quoted morally satisfactory prescriptions in the light of any number of troubling practical cases. First, consider Callahan's claim that we cannot waive our right to life. Callahan does concede that suicide may be such an example, but of course there are many others, including the many forms of self-sacrifice for the sake of others or for the sake of a cause with which human history is replete; acts of self-immolation in protest against war and invasion, self-sacrifice in the name of women's suffrage and so on. I consider talk of 'rights' here confusing; better to talk of moral reasons since our moral evaluation of such cases rests on the degree to which the reasons underpinning such acts amount to a sufficient justification and not whether the acts conform to some absolute ideal. Although Callahan concedes the possibility, I would go further and say there are some compelling examples, where a person is justified in taking or sacrificing their own life:

> Joe is a member of a 'resistance' organisation bent on defeating the forces of a cruel invading army. Joe has sworn absolute obedience to this organisation. Joe is ordered on a mission that will almost certainly result in his death, since he is ordered to kill himself rather than be taken alive. Joe accepts his assignment and takes his own life evading capture.

Consider one possible analysis of this example; Joe does not want to die, he is not nor ever has felt suicidal; equally Joe does not want to be captured and tortured, with the virtually certain consequence that he will 'break' therefore putting his comrades at risk by disclosing information to the enemy. Joe does want to further the cause of the resistance. All things considered Joe willingly accepts his assignment because the cause provides overarching justification. Now this does seem to be an example where an individual waives the right to life and gives authority to another to end that life, and if the mere order to carry out the mission is unconvincing as a life-ending act then consider a further scenario: Joe is injured and a comrade kills him at his request to prevent his capture. Of course, a factor in our judging this whole scenario as justified will hinge crucially on certain other key facts, the 'worthiness' of the cause, for example; however, this does not detract from the general point that *in extremis* such measures are justified, even the waiving of one's right to life and the empowerment of another to take it. Talk of rights, however, is misleading, we should talk rather of the adequacy of the reasons underpinning the act.

There are many other examples in which suicide as an act of self-sacrifice for others shows that this form of killing does not readily fall into the category of *wrongful* killing. Cherry-Garrard's account of Scott's ill-fated polar expedition of 1910 (Cherry-Garrard 1922) is a revealing insight into the ethics of extreme exploration and the sacrifices required. The extreme conditions of such an expedition force the explorer to recognise that:

> Practically any man who undertakes big polar journeys must face the possibility of having to commit suicide to save his companions.
>
> (1922: 537)

The principle of self-sacrifice can therefore even be regarded as a noble act and possibly a morally-required act. The fact that suicide has been justified, even from a Christian ethical perspective, where the suicide is intended in the interests of others, seems to suggest a paradigm example of where deliberately ending a life is both justified and right (Battin 1994).

The reality of suicide as a reasonable, if not required, option in some extreme circumstances is also revealed in the diaries of Scott and those of his party members, who all perished on their return journey from the South Pole. Perhaps the most memorable event is the gesture of Captain Oates who seemingly sacrificed himself by walking out into a blizzard, and certain death, having some days earlier implored his companions to leave him behind. As I have suggested, Oates' gesture was probably one of self-sacrifice, and, as such, in keeping with the convention of morally-justified suicide. Scott's diary, however, also reveals that he ordered the expedition's doctor to make available to each man the means of taking his own life for reasons more ambiguous than the principle of self-sacrifice. Although it is believed that none of the party made use of such contingencies, but had they done so it is interesting to speculate on how we would judge their end? Would we have considered their end less heroic or somehow culpable had they achieved by their own hand what cold and starvation eventually did? I believe that, in the same way as Oates is regarded as a hero and his act seen as one of dignity and courage, we would also regard Scott and his companions in the same light had they taken their opium to achieve an early release.

Although the polar desert is a long way from the hospice, Scott and his companions could be regarded as, in a sense, terminally ill since they had reached a point when their deaths were imminent and inevitable. The issuing of the opium has parallels therefore to assisted suicide; but this is not the point of the example, which is rather to show that our intuitions about the wrongness of killing stand re-examination in the light of real cases. A final case makes a different point. Kyle was interviewed by Magnusson (2002) in his study of euthanasia in Australia. Kyle had been a medic in Vietnam and disclosed the following experience:

> As a medic in Vietnam Kyle practised 'death out of necessity'. 'We got hit one night and had four major burns. It was obvious that two would not survive even in the best of conditions and our chances of getting more than two out in the middle of the monsoons was questionable, so we opted to send two out by helicopter, barely got them out, and then I euthanised the other two with large doses of morphine'.
>
> (Magnusson 2002: 13)

The example is disturbing, but applying the EAPC guidelines as a strict definition of 'moral' categories, we ought to categorize this as a case of murder, whereas I would suggest that our moral intuition is to see this as compassionate killing by necessity.

Citing these examples from outside of the palliative care context is a graphic way of illustrating the point that our intuition that killing is wrong is much more pragmatic than absolute. I accept that, while showing that self-sacrifice and compassionate killing tests our intuitions, it does not move us closer towards a position of accepting a place for these forms of killing in palliative care. This is not my point. What I want to show is that, by acknowledging the pragmatic nature of our moral categories, we can see there is scope for change, moral evolution even, in how we interpret those intuitions. I believe that in medicine, including palliative care, there has been a shift towards accepting some forms of assisting dying that have become so routine, that they are no longer regarded as being in the same moral category as killing. I quote again from Randall and Downie:

> The benefit of alleviating severe distress is considered by patients and carers to outweigh the possible harm by shortening the duration of the terminal illness.
>
> (Randall and Downie 1999: 119)

I shall return to the importance of this pragmatic shift in position in the discussion below.

The argument for self-determination

As I have observed throughout this book, there seems to be some consensus in the West that, on questions concerning what constitutes the best sort of life for an individual, the authority to determine this ought to rest with the person whose life it is. Something akin to this view underpins the liberal concepts of self-determination and respect for autonomy. This marks the point at which axiology, or the theory of the good life, meets ethics. A number of intuitions seem to hold good here, for example, the idea that the best sort of life for a person is a life lived from the 'inside' according to one's own reasons and purposes. In circumstances where we believe it possible to determine objectively what is good for someone else, it still seems reasonable to allow a person to decide for him or herself. At work here is a basic moral belief about what it is to show respect for a person that involves some version of the idea that to show respect for a person is to allow them at least this degree of freedom, even if what this amounts to is the freedom merely to make their own mistakes.

Alongside this basic view runs a number of what might be called 'modifying principles', which are themselves given different weight in different circumstances. The liberal philosopher John Stuart Mill argued a fundamental point, and a foundational one in liberal ethics, when he claimed:

> The only purpose for which power can be rightfully exercised over any member of a civilized community, against his will, is to prevent harm

to others. His own good, either physical or moral, is not a sufficient warrant (1859: 135).

One of the influences the liberal position has had is to engrain a principle of *negative* freedom into the concept of autonomy. Negative freedom means, more generally, a freedom from interference, which is compatible with an equal degree of freedom for others. However, I have argued that the 'rightful exercise of power' does not exclude the reasonable and proper challenge to a person's view of their own good; indeed, most people would expect a doctor or other health professional to challenge a patient's beliefs about what will cure their ailment, where the patient's beliefs are not informed by the evidence. As I have argued, I suggest that is a role which the palliative care community can fulfil, by offering a vision of a better way of dying.

A further modifier to this basic principle of self-determination may also be justified in the interests of a greater common good. There are many examples where such constraints are an accepted part of public life, including where compulsory military service is required or loss of liberty imposed for reasons of public health, as well as the other more minor constraints on liberty that are a necessary part of living within a community. Callahan recognizes the necessity of such constraints on self-determination and, in doing so, argues that AVE falls within the category of actions that ought to be constrained. The problem with Callahan's argument is that we can agree with all of the earlier points of his argument, yet still fail to see why this is the point at which the boundary to self-determination should be drawn unless we had already excepted the conclusion prior to the argument! To press this argument home there are usually two tactics involved; the first is to appeal to absolutes and the second is to appeal to side-effects. I believe that my previous analysis has shown that the wrongness of killing is not a plausible moral absolute. With respect to the bad side-effects, although these have been well discussed in the extensive literature, for example, discussing the side-effects of euthanasia in the Netherlands, I shall consider some of these in my following discussion of palliative care. One issue on which there is near universal agreement within palliative care is the acceptance of death, but the denial of a right to die with assistance. Viewed in the context of the history of palliative care and its underpinning Christian axiology, this stance has the tenor of an objection to voluntary euthanasia that is a theological absolute of the form already described (Oderberg 2000a). Admittedly, it would be going too far to generalize the claim that the whole of modern palliative care shares the same specifically Christian proscription against assisted dying, clearly objections to euthanasia do have a secular basis, a point acknowledged by the palliative care community (Association of Palliative Medicine 1993). My point is rather that given the Christian influence on palliative care, it is reasonable to suppose that the origins of this position are under a similar influence. The significance of this point is that, although autonomy is recognized within palliative care, as an important component of respect for persons, the scope of autonomy is constrained by an over-arching axiology, which in the early development of palliative care took a broadly Christian view of the good life. It is against such a background, I suggest, that the anti-euthanasia stance of palliative care has traditionally been taken. However, as palliative care has evolved into a contemporary medical speciality, then such values have shifted. One influential factor in this shift has been the medicalization of palliative care. Palliative care has therefore become gradually secularized and streamlined with the general secular medical approach to ethics.

Palliative care has and, some might argue, must turn to secular bioethics to support its stance against euthanasia and pro 'good death'. One approach, arguably the dominant one in medical ethics, argues that the principle of respect for autonomy requires a distinction between autonomy as a *liberty* claim and autonomy as a *rights* claim, and thereby argues that respect for autonomy is best understood as a liberty claim that carries no obligation to fulfil positive requests. Although secular ethics influenced by this liberal tradition is pulled in other directions, for example, by patients insisting on their rights and defending their claims by recourse to law. I have suggested that there is a rival approach, one which is grounded in a communitarian axiology, and this is the approach that I have argued is compatible with the ethics and values of palliative care. Axiology concerns the rival theories of the good life and how this ought to be pursued. While liberal ethics presumes there is no good life beyond individual conceptions of the good life, communitarians presume that it is only against a back-ground of a shared conception of the good life can individuals define what is good for them. Pursuing this shared conception requires some limits on individual autonomy, but what exactly those limits are is open to question.

It is against a notion of the good life that certain good making features of the good death are constructed. However, there is a difference between advancing a conception of the good life as an aspiration, and realizing the limitations of what can be achieved in individual cases. There are two ways in which this can fail for individuals. The first is that many people will just not realize the ideal; and recognition of this fact has crept into the palliative care literature. Writers now talk of the 'least worst' or 'good enough' death, of conveying success in terms of the absence of distress or the management of symptoms (Clark and Seymour 1999). The second is more abstract, what I have referred to as the 'endorsement constraint' (Dworkin 1989), it can be put this way: I may live my life to its natural end, and in a way that conforms to the palliative care model, but this may not be a form of living that I value. As Dworkin puts it: 'Value cannot be poured into a life from the outside, it must be generated by the person whose life it is' (1993: 230).

These two failures are significant because they also undermine an important aspiration of palliative care in relation to euthanasia; an aspiration that takes a bold and a weaker form. The bolder aim is one that is evident in some of Cicely Saunders' earliest writing, that palliative care will render euthanasia unnecessary (Saunders 1959). The weaker form of the ambition is that palliative care is the *alternative* to euthanasia. A significant implication of the weaker aspiration is the possibility of palliative care existing alongside assisted dying; a possibility, as I shall argue, that is compatible both with palliative care and the communitarian approach I have described.

The bold strategy, I believe, will fail for the reasons that I have already given. Even though I also believe that most people with a terminal illness would benefit from palliative care, which cannot relieve suffering in all cases and has so far shown itself very limited in its application outside of the cancer context. The second point is more significant, that is, even if palliative care were broadly successful in controlling symptoms and maintaining quality of life, some individuals, possibly only very few, would still not value living to their 'natural' death and would therefore prefer some form of assisted dying.

Gordijn and Janssens (2000) offer an argument that could be seen as a response to this latter point. They argue that a decision for euthanasia made at a time of pain and suffering could not be autonomous in any full sense and, therefore, the request should be denied as that of an non-autonomous (incompetent?) request (Gordijn and Janssens 2000: 44). However, I find this tactic implausible, since it may be empirically false, but more significantly, it is also conceptually problematic. Their criticism requires too stringent a criterion for autonomy. This is not to say that people's capacity for making autonomous decisions is never affected by their health or other circumstances. What their argument does show is that, when one is concerned about the competence of a person's decisions then we ought to carefully assess and clearly establish the degree of impairment to a person's capacity. Capacity, as has been frequently observed, may differ with respect to the complexity of the decision, the timing and circumstances. It is therefore reasonable to suppose that some terminally ill people will lack autonomy and some will not. However, questions about *an* individual's capacity are quite separate from the question of whether a request for assisted dying ought to be respected on the grounds of the principle of respect for autonomy. If autonomy is relevant to the practice of palliative care and at least some terminally ill people are autonomous, then a further argument is needed to justify the limits imposed upon certain wishes.

What this also points to, as in the many cases of moral debate about the human good, is that there is a need for sound empirical evidence to support some of the more abstract arguments. Of course evidence does not make arguments, but evidence does provide reasons. The English House of Lords

Select Committee on the Assisted Dying for the Terminally Ill Bill (ADTI House of Lords 2005) heard a range of evidence, some of which was conceptual and some empirical. Arguments that attack the wrongness of euthanasia and assisted dying often draw upon empirical evidence to point to the bad side-effects of these interventions, yet there is also empirical evidence of benefit. Swarte *et al.* (2003) reports on the effects of euthanasia on bereavement. Although they report their findings with caveats, they say that the bereaved family and friends of cancer patients who died by euthanasia, coped better with the death than those bereaved through natural death. Some of the benefits they cite include being able to plan for the end, being able to prepare and having an opportunity to say goodbye. They conclude: 'These results should not be interpreted as a plea for euthanasia, but as a plea for the same level of care and openness in all patients who are terminally ill' (2003: 329).

The authors' appeal that their work should not be seen as arguing in favour of euthanasia is actually undermined by their own evidence. I earlier made the point that even the best of palliative care cannot promise to give people a good death. It is therefore not only possible, but highly probable that assisted dying in some circumstances will be more effective at achieving the goals of the good death because there is a willingness to engineer this end, rather than to leave it to the uncertainty of chance.

It has been my observation throughout this book that palliative care has been increasingly willing to manage actively the parameters of the good death. I believe that, even though the majority of the palliative care community is a long way from accepting such a proposition, the way to realize the 'good death' is to begin to accept the possible compatibility of palliative care with assisted dying methods. The wider use and acceptability of palliative sedation is perhaps an indication of a willingness to take the first step in this direction. The next step ought to be the acceptance of assisted suicide in a form outlined in the ADTI Bill (House of Lords 2005) or by some similar reform of legislation.

Palliative care: assisting the good death?

The idea that euthanasia and assisted dying may be compatible with, indeed, should be an integral part of, palliative care is not a new idea [Heintz 1994, *Federatie Palliatieve Zorg Vlaanderen* (FPZV) 2003]. However, in the final section of this chapter I wish to expand upon this claim within the context of the arguments that I have made throughout this book. I wish, in particular, to show how this claim is consistent with the communitarian axiology of palliative care. I suggest that, if the palliative care community controlled this intervention, then there would be less chance of abuse, more chance that people would realize the benefits of palliative care and live to die a natural death. Of course, these are empirical claims and before a step is taken towards verifying such claims there is a need for robust arguments and I shall now attempt to provide some of these. The WHO (2002) definition claims that palliative care: 'intends neither to hasten nor postpone death' and this may be seen as a reiteration of the traditional palliative stance against euthanasia or assisted dying. Randall and Downie (2006) offer a well argued and effective criticism of this statement, which is flawed in many ways. Not the least of these is that a short sentence can never hope to provide an adequate philosophy for what is a highly complex and controversial set of issues. Randall and Downie go on to offer their own analysis of how this aspect of end-of-life care should be approached, and in doing so they clarify and restate what they see as the standard medical ethical and medico-legal position within which palliative care ought to operate. I entirely endorse their view that it is, and ought to be, a goal of palliative care to employ measures that might prolong life, which is of good quality and valued by the patient, during the phase prior to imminent death. More significantly, they also endorse a view that demonstrates the shift in palliative care values from an absolute belief in the sanctity of life to a pragmatic acceptance that hastening death is justified. They of course acknowledge that the concept of 'hastening death' is itself ambiguous and they attempt to clarify their own position, first, with regard to withholding and withdrawing treatment and, second with regard to relieving suffering. On the first point they state:

For instance, when life-prolonging treatments such as artificial nutrition and hydration are removed from patients in the persistent vegetative state, or artificial ventilation is removed from stable but unconscious ventilator-dependent patients, it is overwhelmingly likely that death will follow, and so some people consider that such a withdrawal of life-prolonging treatment actually causes the patient's death. They therefore think that it should be considered morally and legally to be the cause of the patient's death. Legally, causing the patient's death is one of the two conditions for murder.

On the other hand, we would wish to argue that the patient's death is caused by the underlying failure of essential organ function ... the fundamental cause of death is the patient's condition, not the withdrawal of treatment, which should be regarded as *incidental*. Death would have been caused by the pathological conditions of PVS or inability to breathe ... if in these situations there is no reasonable hope of recovery of consciousness or ability to breathe, further life-sustaining treatment cannot confer benefit and therefore it is not in the patient's interests to continue it. When it is removed the body's own causality results in death.

(Randall and Downie 2006: 109, emphasis added)

I do not wish to spend too long on the analysis of this kind of argument that already occupies an extensive body of literature. I do, however, wish to make a number of observations. First, with regard to the extract I have quoted, I consider this to be one of the clearest statements of the 'standard' position. However, in the same way that the WHO statement disguises significant complexity, then so too does Randall and Downie's statement. The first thing to note is that the example they use is that of a permanently unconscious person, but in the palliative care context withholding and withdrawing does not exclusively occur with permanently unconscious individuals. Furthermore, if we consider a *conscious* person who has permanently lost the ability to breathe then the context is still further complicated. Ms B (Boyd 2002), it will be recalled, was conscious, but had permanent paralysis including the inability to breathe. Controversially, Ms B was not 'dying', indeed, in the view of many, she had the prospect of living a worthwhile life. The point is that Ms B did not foresee her prospects positively and believed that it would be better if she were to die. In order to achieve what she believed was in her best interests she needed assistance to remove the ventilator which kept her alive. Now to regard the removal of the ventilator as 'incidental', as Randall and Downie imply, is to deceive by understatement. A major consideration in Ms B's case was the status of the act of removal and its causal role in her eventual death. If the removal of the ventilator was merely *incidental*, playing no causal role in her death, merely preventing her death by 'natural causes' then this should have been enough to satisfy those doctors who so strongly objected to performing this act. The 'no causal role' argument might appear easier to accept in the case of a PVS patient, but it seems highly counter-intuitive in the case of a person in Ms B's situation. On Randall and Downie's analysis admitting a causal role entails the possibility of classifying such 'acts' as murder yet we are highly reluctant to describe such outcomes as occurred in the case of Ms B as either 'murder' or 'suicide'. In both moral and legal terms these kinds of death occupy an ambiguous category. To deny this is to deny the very complexity that Randall and Downie are seeking to avoid. I suggest that the honest approach is to accept that it is right to cause death in some circumstances, and these should be regarded as justified or 'appropriate' killings and not murder; this would, of course, entail a change in the law. This brings me to my second point; the palliative care community already accepts that making a causal contribution towards a person's death is both ethical and required by good practice. The circumstance in which this occurs within palliative care is in response to intractable suffering; and again I quote from Randall and Downie:

> However, there are clinical situations in which a treatment given with the aim of relieving distressing symptoms at the end of life may actually have other effects which may make death occur earlier than it

would have done without the treatment. It is important to remember that such treatments are not the cause of death entirely, but in the context of the patient's advanced illness and frailty death may occur earlier than without the treatment.

(Randall and Downie 2006: 113)

I take this passage to state that making a causal contribution to or *assisting* a patient's death is an ethical and appropriate part of palliative care. Randall and Downie later summarize their point in the context of their proposed new philosophy of palliative care:

Health care practitioners may justifiably hasten death as a foreseen but not intended effect of treatment whose aim is the treatment of pain and distress at the end of life.

(Randall and Downie 2006: 221)

Randall and Downie, as part of their justification for accepting the validity of hastening death, place emphasis on the role of intention and, in doing so, utilize the traditional Doctrine of Double Effect. However, as I argued in chapter 5, if intention is construed as a 'mental state', a thought in the mind of the doctor, then this is a fragile and subjective criterion on which to base such an important distinction as that between murder and care. My suggestion that intention should be an 'external' criterion based upon objective standards of practice is a much more robust way of making the point. I would therefore modify Randall and Downie's statement to read that 'health care practitioners may justifiably hasten death in the context of appropriate treatment for pain and distress at the end of life' where 'appropriate' is judged on the quality of the clinical decision, and the context in which it is made. The thrust of my argument is that 'hastening death', in Randall and Downie's sense is morally equivalent to justifiably assisting dying. In summary, my point is that if death can be justifiably caused by means which are slow and indirect there is no moral difference between this and employing means that are faster and more direct.

Of course, Randall and Downie would not accept this conclusion, but neither do I accept that their argument based on syllogism, offered both within the context of their book and as written evidence to the House of Lords (ADTI Bill 2005), is a valid rejoinder. Their argument is expressed in this form:

Major premise: Morally indistinguishable cases should not be treated differently by law.
Minor premise: Acts of letting die are morally indistinguishable from acts of mercy killing or euthanasia.
Conclusion: Therefore the law should not treat acts of mercy killing or euthanasia differently from acts of letting die.

While the conclusion does follow logically from both premises, we would contend that the premises are seriously flawed and so the conclusion based on them should be rejected.

(Randall and Downie 2006: 115)

It should, of course, be noted that while the minor premise addresses acts of letting die, my own argument concerns hastening and assisting death. However, I suggest that the minor premise could be substituted by the following premise: acts that foresee the hastening of death are morally indistinguishable from acts of assisting death. On the basis of this modification Randall and Downie's criticism might be seen to hold good against my argument. However, I would like to make a number of points in defence. To begin with, I would argue that this syllogistic form of reasoning begs the question concerning what is at stake here. For one, I am not convinced that advocates of the moral equivalence argument are making a strictly *logical* claim about synonymous terms. I do not believe that the claim '*x* is *morally* equivalent to *y*' is to claim that *x* is *synonymous* with *y*. Rather, it is to argue something less precise. I suggest that my argument, and similar moral equivalence claims can be understood as asserting that: Given the range of acts that might be said to deliberately assist death (*x*) then *x* is, morally speaking, much more like the range of acts said to foresee the hastening of death (*y*), than *x* is like a straightforward case of murder (*z*). So in this context the claim that $x = y + x \neq z$ are not logical claims, but plausible empirical moral claims, that invite us to envisage undergoing a transition in our moral thinking by weighing the various reasons for one position over another. Implicit in the argument is also a normative argument for the revision of the law. The claim about what the law ought to do rests upon a deeper argument that certain legal constructions force us to apply a framework of distinctions, which is not adequate for our moral needs. Moral needs that are themselves evolving and changing. The implication therefore is that if we revise the law to reflect our reasoned moral beliefs then those beliefs will not be constrained by too blunt a legal instrument.

My point, therefore, is that since some forms of hastening death are accepted as part of a justifiable clinical approach, then it is within the scope of palliative care to incorporate other more explicit and direct means of hastening death.

Hastening death and palliative care values

How could forms of hastening death including euthanasia and assisted suicide be deemed compatible with palliative care given its long-standing opposition to such interventions? The approach I suggest to this reconciliation is to regard euthanasia and assisted suicide as being on a continuum with the use of sedation in palliative contexts. In this regard such extreme measures might be seen as an option of last resort. I suggest that the concepts of appropriateness and proportionality could be applied so that only the terminally ill person would receive assistance in dying, and whose desire for death was refractory to receiving specialist palliative care.

I therefore suggest that integrating legal options for assisted dying into palliative care would incorporate what has been called a 'palliative filter'. The concept of a palliative filter has received most recent attention in the discussions that preceded the legalization of euthanasia in Belgium (Broeckaert and Janssens 2002). In the period prior to drawing up legislation, the FPZV conducted a series of debates, consultations, interviews and symposia including lobbying politicians advocating the Bill. The FPZV were anxious to include a 'palliative filter' within the Bill to ensure that patients requesting euthanasia could be suitably assessed in order to ensure that their consent to euthanasia was premised upon the fullest consideration of their options, and an expert palliative care assessment of the patient's symptoms and mental state. This, it was suggested should take the form of a palliative care assessment prior to any decision regarding euthanasia. The form of filter that I am suggesting is that the request for assisted dying should only be considered once the patient has been in receipt of specialist palliative care for some time. In suggesting this form of 'palliative filter' I am drawing on a concept derived from ideals expressed much earlier in the history of palliative care.

Opposition to assisted dying has been consistently and clearly voiced by Cicely Saunders, yet the idea that palliative care may be an alternative to and preventive of euthanasia also suggests the possibility that receiving specialist palliative care is the most effective form of 'palliative filter'. To illustrate my point, I will draw on an experience described by Saunders in her letter to Dr A. Sickel in the Netherlands:

> 31 May 1972 Thank you for your most interesting paper. I was particularly interested in your comments on loneliness. I am afraid that I do not agree with you at the end where you suggest that we may have come to the place of active euthanasia ... Perhaps I could summarize a conversation I had with a patient last weekend. Sister has told me about your conversation [a request to end her life]. You know I cannot give you an overdose but suppose for the sake of argument I could. Would you like me to do it now? The instant response was 'No, not now ...' I think that this sort of request is so often near the end and comes from the utter weariness which we can help. Never when I have asked 'Do you want it now' have I been given the answer 'Yes.'
>
> (Clark 2002: 152)

I have used this example from Saunders' writing because I believe that it gives a working example of how the 'palliative filter' I envisage might work;

and I shall specify some of the features I suggest are implicit here. One thing the example shows is how a skilled and experienced carer is able to engage in a conversation about euthanasia with a patient. It also implies that a patient who has actually had experience of palliative care is informed and not merely theoretically so, of how palliative care may benefit them. Also knowing that the option of assisted dying is there, may itself be reassuring without having to make use of the option. Of course, the difference is that I am advocating that the option may actually be used should the patient say 'Yes'. Resorting to assisted dying within palliative care must be, in my view, subject to the model argued for in chapter 5, that the patient's symptoms, physical or existential, are refractory to specialist palliative care.

The incorporation of assisted death options within palliative care is entirely consistent with the communitarian axiology within which I have argued; the contemporary palliative care alternative is rooted. Palliative care offers a vision of the good death and it is within this context that certain constraints upon individual choices and autonomy may be justified in terms of requiring a person to experience the palliative care way. However, unlike Hurst and Mauron (2006), I am not only arguing that there are common values between palliative care and the advocates of assisted dying. I am arguing that the measures used to assist dying are morally consistent extensions of the measures routinely used within palliative care to manipulate the process of dying along its best course.

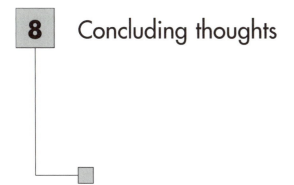

8 Concluding thoughts

Despite the death defying technologies of the modern age, it remains a certainty that we will pass into death's dominion. However, the manner and timing of our death is something over which we can aspire to have some control. Palliative care has strived to offer the hope that the worst of our fears about death will not be realized and that our dying may be as worthwhile as any other aspect of our lives. To this end palliative care, from its origins in the modern hospices, has endeavoured to intervene actively so as to engineer the conditions under which the best possible death for the individual may be realized. In this book, I set out to explore the concepts and values which underpin this endeavour and to offer an argument as to the direction in which palliative care ought to evolve.

I began this book by reflecting on the nature of ethics and value in general. I offered a critique of some of the standard and dominant ethical theories, and I argued that a pragmatic approach to ethics is one that is more suited to reflection upon ethics generally, but palliative care and end of life issues particularly. The pragmatic approach recognises that habits and practises are primarily the vehicle for moral action. To this extent I agree with Randall and Downie (2006) that a philosophy of palliative care must influence the habits and practises of palliative carers. However, we also live in a state of flux, new technologies, a mobile society and shifting social values. Because pragmatic ethics is dynamic, requiring iterative reflection, it is especially suited to use within a practical discipline like palliative care, which seeks to be relevant in changing contexts. My purpose, therefore, was to write a book that combined a philosophical exploration of beliefs and values with a practical consideration of the challenges we face at the end-of-life. The readers will no doubt judge whether I have been successful in that purpose.

In my analysis of the history and evolution of palliative care, I was inspired not only to offer an accurate historical account, although this has been done much better by far more knowledgeable scholars, but also to render explicit the concepts and values that drove that evolution. The belief that there was a better way of dying, than contemporary society offered, inspired the early hospices. The idea that this could best be offered within a community, in a special place, quickly gave way to the knowledge that those ideals and principles could apply wherever a dying person found themselves or preferred to be. Palliative care has a vision for how the good death might be realized, a vision born out of human wisdom and practical know how. Palliative care philosophy aspired to combine scientifically robust treatment of symptoms with a team approach to offering holistic care, including spiritual and psycho-social care of the patient and their family. This approach was to be delivered, ideally, in a place of the patient's choosing and in an atmosphere of open awareness knowing that the patient was terminally ill and would die.

The emergence of specialist palliative care and its focus on palliative medicine brought advances in evidence-based practice, making inroads into the management of symptoms. However, the medicalization of palliative care has created tensions. Randall and Downie (1999, 2006) have argued that the future for palliative care lies in conforming to the model of medicine, and their revised philosophy of palliative care is clearly informed by the medical model. Although this shift may secure both status and resources for palliative medicine, it may be at the price of the palliative care vision that there is a better way of living and dying.

The issue of what individuals have a right to expect for themselves, in terms of the resources to achieve a good death, is a persistent theme. Randall and Downie note that the emergence of consumer autonomy is a threat both to palliative care and to medicine. They argue that there are trends in palliative care that encourage this model, whereas the liberal ethics of medicine restricts the rights of the patient to the right of non-interference. Liberalism, however, cannot offer the vision of a better alternative that is so distinctive of the palliative care philosophy. I have argued that, in contrast to liberal and consumer autonomy, palliative care philosophy is consistent with a communitarian approach. This locates autonomy within a broader context of respect for persons, attempting to reconcile the restrictions on individual autonomy against the vision of a better way of living and dying. The challenge for this vision is that it must keep pace with social change, while maintaining the foil of the palliative care alternative.

For all that is valuable in palliative care, I have also argued in favour of extending the control that individuals are permitted to have over the quality of their dying and death, including assisted dying. This is why I am cautiously in favour of legislative change. I have argued that the Law ought to permit assisted dying restricted to the terminal phases of a condition in circumstances where the person has passed through the 'palliative filter' and received the attention of specialist palliative care.

Why do I favour the restricted approach? The real plight of people, so frequently reported in the media forces one to think about the issues they raise. One of these issues is the problem of a still capable and competent individual attempting to foresee their own best interests in circumstances for which they have no experience, and only their worst fears to provoke the imagination. This is understandable, since many of us who believe ourselves to be a long way from our own deaths find it difficult to imagine that we might grow to peacefully accept the changes in one's mind and body that accompany the imminent approach of death. I have argued that palliative care has long accepted that we should aspire to greater control over the aspects of dying that may make it better or worse. I conclude, therefore, that palliative care can and must accept that extending this control to assisting death is both right and consistent with palliative care values.

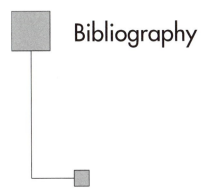

Bibliography

Ahmedzai, S. (1996) Making a success out of life's failure. *Progress in Palliative Care*, 4: 1–3.

Aries, P. (1976) *Western Attitudes Towards Death: From the Middle Ages to the Present*. London: Marion Boyars.

Aristotle. (1925) *Nicomachean Ethics*. Trans. W.D. Ross. Oxford: Clarendon Press.

Armstrong, D. (1995) The rise of surveillance medicine. *Social Science and Medicine*, 24: 651–7.

Ashby, M.A. and Stoffell, B. (1991) Therapeutic ratio and defined phases: proposal of ethical framework for palliative care. *British Medical Journal*, 302: 1322–4.

Association of Palliative Medicine (1993) Submission from the ethics group of the Association of Palliative Medicine of Great Britain and Ireland to The Select Committee of the House of Lords on Medical Ethics. 1F/PJH/3/Lords.

Bassnet, I. (2002) Will to live wins over right to die. *The Observer*, 24 March.

Battin, P. M. (1994) *The Least Worst Death*. New York, NY: Oxford University Press.

Bauman, Z. (1997) *Post Modernity and its Discontents*. Oxford: Polity Press.

Beauchamp, T.L. and Childress, V.F. (2003) *Principles of Biomedical Ethics*, revised edn. New York, NY: Oxford University Press.

Bentham, J. (1789) *An Introduction to the Principles of Morals and Legislation*. Oxford: Oxford University Press.

Billings, J.A. and Block, S.D. (1996) Slow Euthanasia, *Journal of Palliative Care*, 12(4): 38–41.

Billings, J.A. (1998) What is palliative care? *Journal of Palliative Medicine*, 1(1): 73–81.

Biswas, B. (1993) The medicalization of dying, in: D. Clark (ed.) *The Future for Palliative Care*. Buckingham: Open University Press.

Blustein, J. (1993) The family in medical decision-making, *Hastings Centre Report*, May-June, 23: 6–13.

Boddington, P. and Podpadec, T. (1992) Measuring quality of life in theory and in practice: a dialogue between philosophical and psychological approaches, *Bioethics*, 6(3): 201–217.

Bowling, A. (1995) *Measuring Disease: A Review of Disease Specific Quality of Life Measurement Scales*. Buckingham: Association of Palliative Medicine/Open University Press.

Boyd, K.M. (1995) The development of home care in the UK. *Palliative Care Today*, 4(4): 46–7.

Boyd, K.M. (2002) Mrs Pretty and Ms B, *Journal of Medical Ethics*, 28: 211–2.

Bradshaw, A. (1996) The spiritual dimension of hospice: the secularization of an ideal. *Social Science and Medicine*, 43: 409–19.

Brock, D. (1993) Quality of life measures in health care and medical ethics in: M. Nussbaum and A. Sen (eds.) *The Quality of Life*. Oxford: Clarendon Press, 95–132.

Brody, H. (1996) Commentary on Billings and Block's 'Slow Euthanasia', *Journal of Palliative Care*, 12(4): 38–41.

Broeckaert, B. (2000) Palliative sedation defined or why and when terminal sedation is not euthanasia, abstract 1st Congress RDPC, December, Berlin (Germany), *Journal of Pain and Symptom Management*, 20(6): S58.

Broeckaert, B. (2002) Palliative sedation: ethical aspects in: C. Gastmans (ed.) *Between Technology and Humanity, the Impact of Technology on Health Care Ethics*. Leuven: University Press, 239–55.

Broeckaert, B. and Nunez-Olarte, J.M. (2002) Sedation in palliative care: facts and concepts in: H. ten Have and D. Clark (eds) *The Ethics of Palliative Care: European Perspectives*. Buckingham: Open University Press, 166–80.

Broeckaert, B. and Janssens, R. (2005) Palliative care and euthanasia: Belgian and Dutch perspectives in: P. Schotsmans and T. Meulenbergs (eds) *Euthanasia and Palliative Care in the Low Countries*. Leuven: Peeters, 35—70.

Buxton, M. and Ashby, J. (1988) The time trade-off approach to health state evaluation in: G. Teeling Smith (ed.) *Measuring Health: A Practical Approach*. London: John Wiley and Sons Ltd, 69–87.

Callahan, D. (1992) When self-determination runs amok. *Hastings Centre Report*, 22(2): 52–5.

Callahan, D. (1993) *The Troubled Dream of Life: Living with Mortality*. New York, NY: Simon and Schuster.

Cherny, N.I. (1998) Sedation in response to refractory existential distress: walking the fine line. *Journal of Pain and Symptom Management*, 16: 404–6.

Cherny, N.I. and Portenoy, R.K. (1994) Sedation in the management of refractory symptoms: guidelines for evaluation and treatment. *Journal of Palliative Care*, 10: 31–38.

Cherry-Garrard, A. (1922) *The Worst Journey in The World*. London: Picador.

Clark, D. (1993) Wither the hospices? in: D. Clark (ed.) *The Future for Palliative Care*. Buckingham: Open University Press.

Clark, D. (1998) An annotated bibliography of the publications of Cicely Saunders – 1: 1958–1967. *Palliative Medicine*, 12: 181–93.

Clark, D. (1999a) An annotated bibliography of the publications of Cicely Saunders – 2: 1968–1977. *Palliative Medicine*, 13: 485–501.

Clark, D. (1999b) Cradled to the grave? Preconditions for the hospice movement in the UK 1948–1967. *Mortality*, 4: 225–47.

Clark, D. (2002a) *Cicely Saunders: Founder of the Hospice Movement. Selected Letters 1959–1999.* Oxford: Oxford University Press.

Clark, D. (2002b) Between hope and acceptance: the medicalization of dying. *British Medical Journal,* 324: 904–7.

Clark, D. (2006) The development of palliative medicine in the UK and Ireland in: E. Bruera, I. Higginson, C. Ripamonti, and C. von Gunten (eds) *Textbook of Palliative Medicine.* London: Hodder Arnold, 3–9.

Clark, D., ten Have, H. and Janssens, R. (2002) Palliative care service developments in seven European countries in: H. ten Have and D. Clark (eds) *The Ethics of Palliative Care: European Perspectives.* Buckingham: Open University Press. 34–51.

Clark, D. and Seymour, J. (1999) *Reflections on Palliative Care.* Buckingham: Open University Press.

Clouser, K.D. and Gert, B. (1999) A critique of principlism. *Journal of Medicine and Philosophy,* 15 (2): 219–36.

Comby, M.C. and Filbet, M. (2005) The demand for euthanasia in palliative care units: a prospective study in seven units of the 'Rhône-Alpes' region. *Journal of Palliative Medicine,* 19: 587–93.

Conrad, P. (1992) Medicalization and social control. *Annual Review of Sociology,* 18: 209–32.

Conroy, S.P., Luxton, T., Dingwall, R., Harwood, R.H. and Gladman, J.R.F. (2006) Cardiopulmonary resuscitation in continuing care settings: time for a rethink? *British Medical Journal,* 332: 479–82.

Copp, G. (1998) A review of current theories of dying. *Journal of Advanced Nursing,* 28(2): 382–90.

Craig, G.M. (1994) On withholding nutrition and hydration in the terminally ill: has palliative medicine gone too far? *Journal of Medical Ethics,* 20(3): 139–43.

Department of Health (2000) *The Cancer Plan.* London: Department of Health.

Department of Health/The Welsh Office (1995) *A Policy Framework for Developing Cancer Services.* London: HMSO.

Dignity in Dying (2006) *Dignity in Dying: The Report.* London.

Doyal, L. (2006) The futility of opposing the legalisation of non-voluntary and voluntary euthanasia in: S. McLean (ed.) *First Do No Harm.* Aldershot: Ashgate.

Doyle, D., Hanks, G.W.C. and MacDonald, N. (1993) Introduction in: D. Doyle, G.W.C. Hanks and N. MacDonald (eds) *Oxford Textbook of Palliative Medicine.* Oxford: Oxford University Press.

Dresser, R. (1995) Dworkin on dementia: elegant theory questionable policy. *Hastings Centre Report,* 25(6): 32–8.

Dunlop, R.J., Ellershaw, J.E., Baines, M.J., Sykes, N. and Saunders, C.M. (1995) On withholding nutrition and hydration in the terminally ill: has palliative medicine gone to far? A reply. *Journal of Medical Ethics,* 21: 141–3.

Dworkin, R. (1986) Autonomy and the demented self. *Milbank Quarterly,* 64 (Suppl. 2): 4–16.

Dworkin, G. (1988) *The Theory and Practice of Autonomy.* Cambridge MA: Cambridge University Press.

Dworkin, R. (1989) Liberal community. *California Law Review,* 77(3): 479–504.

Dworkin, R. (1993) *Life's Dominion: An Argument about Abortion, Euthanasia and Individual Freedom.* New York, NY: Alfred A Knopf.

Ellershaw, J.E. (2002) Clinical pathways for care of the dying - an innovation to disseminate clinical excellence. *Journal of Palliative Medicine*, 5(4): 617–23.

Ellershaw, J.E., Smith, C., Overill, S., Walker, S.E. and Aldridge, J. (2001) Care of the dying: setting standards for symptom control in the last 48 hours of life. *Journal of Pain and Symptom Management*, 21(1): 12–7.

Ellershaw, J.E. and Ward, C. (2003) Care of the dying patient: the last hours or days of life. *British Medical Journal*, 326: 30–4.

Ellershaw, J.E. and Wilkinson, S. (2003) *Care of the Dying: A Pathway to Excellence*. Oxford: Oxford University Press.

Jack, B., Gambles, M., Murphy, D. and Ellershaw, J.E. (2003) Nurses' perceptions of the Liverpool Care Pathway for the dying patient in the acute hospital setting. *International Journal of Palliative Nursing*, 9(9): 375–81.

Evans. S, (2004) Whose life is it anyway? *Healthcare News Brief.* London: Hempsons Solicitors Autumn: 1.

Farsides, C.C.S. (1998) Autonomy and its implications for palliative care: a Northern European perspective. *Palliative Medicine*, 12: 147–51.

Federatie Palliatieve Zorg Vlaanderen (Flemish Palliative Care Federation) (2003) *Dealing with Euthanasia and other Forms of Medically Assisted Death*.

Field, D. (1994) Palliative medicine and the medicalization of death. *European Journal of Cancer Care*, 3: 58–62.

Field, D. (1996) Awareness and modern dying. *Mortality*, 1: 255–66.

Field, D., Hockey, J. and Small, N. (1997) *Death Gender and Ethnicity*. London: Routledge.

Gastmans, C., Lemiengre, J., van der Wal, G., Schotsmans, P. and Dierckx, de Casterl'e B. (2006) *Prevalence and Content of Written Ethics Policies on Euthanasia in Catholic Healthcare Institutions in Belgium (Flanders).* Health Policy 76: 169–78.

Geddes, L. (1973) On the intrinsic wrongness of killing innocent people. *Analysis*, 34: 16–9.

General Medical Council (2002) *Withholding and Withdrawing Life-Prolonging Treatment: Good Practice in Decision-Making.* London: GMC.

Gillick, M.R. (2005) Rethinking the central dogma of palliative care. *Journal of Palliative Medicine*, 8(5): 909–13.

Glover, J. (1984) *Causing Death and Saving Lives*. 1st edn. London: Penguin Books.

Glover, J. (1989) *The Philosophy and Psychology of Personal Identity*. Middlesex: Penguin.

Gordijn, B. and Janssens, R. (2000) The prevention of euthanasia through palliative care: new developments in the Netherlands. *Patient Education and Counselling*, 41: 35–46.

Gostin, L.O. (2005) Ethics, the constitution and the dying process, the case of Theresa Marie Schiavo. *Journal of the American Medical Association*, 293: 2403–7.

Gracia, D. (2002) From conviction to responsibility in palliative care ethics in: H. ten Have and D. Clark (eds) *The Ethics of Palliative Care: European Perspectives.* Buckingham: Open University Press, 87–105.

Griffin, J. (1986) *Well-being: Its Meaning, Measurement and Moral Importance.* Oxford: Oxford University Press.

Grisso, T. and Appelbaum, P.S. (1998) *Assessing Competence to Consent to*

Treatment: A Guide for Physicians and Other Health Care Professionals. New York, NY: Oxford University Press.

Hamilton, J. (1995) Dr. Balfour Mount and the cruel irony of our care for the dying. *Canadian Medical Association Journal,* 153(3): 334–6.

Hardwig, J. (1990) What about the family? *Hastings Centre Report,* 10 (2): 5–10.

Harris, J. (1983) In vitro fertilization: the ethical issues (I). *The Philosophical Quarterly,* 132: 217–37.

Harris, J. (1985) *The Value of Life: An Introduction to Medical Ethics.* London: Routledge and Kegan Paul.

Harris, J. (1995) Euthanasia and the value of life, in: J. Keown (ed.) *Euthanasia Examined: Ethical, Clinical and Legal Perspectives.* Cambridge MA: Cambridge University Press, 6–22.

Harris, J. (1999) The Concept of the person and the value of life. *Kennedy Institute of Ethics Journal,* 9(4): 293–308.

Hart, B., Sainsbury, P. and Short, S. (1998) Whose dying? A sociological critique of the 'good death'. *Mortality,* 3: 65–77.

Häyry, M. (2004) Another look at dignity. *Cambridge Quarterly of Healthcare Ethics,* 13: 7–14.

Heintz, A.P.M. (1994) Euthanasia: can be part of good terminal care. *British Medical Journal,* 308: 1656.

Henderson, V. (1960) *Basic Principles of Nursing Care.* Geneva: International Council of Nurses.

Higginson, I. (1997) Palliative and terminal care in: A. Stevens and J. Rafferty (eds) *Health Care Needs Assessment.* Oxford: Radcliffe Medical Press.

Holm, S. (1995) Not just autonomy – the principles of American biomedical ethics. *Journal of Medical Ethics,* 21: 332–8.

House of Lords (2005a) *Select Committee on the Assisted Dying for the Terminally Ill Bill. Vol. I: Report.* London: The Stationery Office Limited.

House of Lords (2005b) *Select Committee on the Assisted Dying for the Terminally Ill Bill. Vol. II: Evidence.* London: The Stationery Office Limited.

Hughes, G.H.L. (1960) *Peace at the Last. A Survey of Terminal Care in the United Kingdom.* London: The Calouste Gulbenkian Foundation.

Hurst, S. and Mauron, A. (2006) The ethics of palliative care and euthanasia: exploring common values. *Palliative Medicine,* 20(2): 107–12.

Huxtable, R. (2004) Get out of jail free? The doctrine of double effect in English law. *Palliative Medicine,* 18(1) 62–8.

Illich, I. (1976) *Limits to Medicine. Medical Nemesis: The Expropriation of Health.* London: Penguin.

James, N. and Field, D. (1992) The routinization of hospice: charisma and bureaucratization. *Social Science and Medicine,* 34: 1363.

Janssens, R. (2001) *Palliative Care: Concepts and Ethics.* Nijmegen: Nijmegen University Press.

Joint National Cancer Survey Committee of the Marie Curie memorial and The Queen's Institute of District Nursing (1952) *A Report on a National Survey Concerning Patients with Cancer Nursed at Home.* London: Marie Curie Memorial.

Jonsen, A. (1990) *The New Medicine and the Old Ethics.* Cambridge, MA: Harvard University Press.

Kant, I. (1786) *Groundwork for the Metaphysics of Morals.* Trans. J.J. Paton

(1964),New York, NY: Harper and Row.

Kearney, M. (1992) Palliative medicine – just another speciality? *Palliative Medicine*, 6: 39–46.

Kearney, M. (2000) *A Place of Healing: Working with Suffering in Living and Dying*. Oxford: Oxford University Press.

Kelly, G. (1951) 'The Duty to Preserve Life', *Theological Studies*, 12 December: 550.

Kenny, A. (1992) *Aristotle on the Perfect Life*. Oxford: Clarendon Press.

Kirkwood, T. (2000) *Time of Our Lives*. London: Phoenix.

Krakauer, J. (1997) *Into Thin Air*. London: Macmillan.

Kubler-Ross, E. (1969) *On Death and Dying*. London: Tavistock.

Kuhse, H. (1987) *The Sanctity of Life Doctrine in Medicine: A Critique*. Oxford: Oxford University Press.

Kuhse, H. (2002) Response to Ronal M. Perkin and David B. Resnik: the agony of trying to match sanctity of life and patient-centred medical care. *Journal of Medical Ethics*, 28: 270–2.

Kuhse, H. (2004) Why terminal sedation is no solution to the voluntary euthanasia debate in: T. Tännsjö (ed.) *Terminal Sedation*. Dordrecht, Kluwer Academic Press, 57–70.

Kurland, A. (1985) LSD in the supportive care of the terminally ill cancer patients. *Journal of Psychoactive Drugs*, 17(4): 279–90.

Kymlicka, W. (1990) *Contemporary Political Philosophy: An introduction*. Oxford: Clarendon Press.

LaFollette, H. (2000) Pragmatic ethics in: H. LaFolletee (ed.) *The Blackwell Guide to Ethical Theory*. Oxford: Blackwell Publishers, 400–19.

Levinas, E. (1989) Ethics as first philosophy in: S. Hand (ed.) *The Levinas Reader*. Oxford: Blackwell Publications, 75–87.

Locke, J. (1976) *An essay Concerning Human Understanding*. London: Dent.

Lynn, J, and Adamson, D.M. (2003) *Living Well at the End of Life. Adapting Health-Care to Serious Chronic Illness in Old Age*. Washington, WA: Rand Health.

MacIntyre, A. (1981) *After Virtue: A Study in Moral Theory*. London: Duckworth.

MacIntyre, A. (1999) *Dependent Rational Animals: Why Humans Need the Virtues*. Chicago, IL: Carus Publishing Company.

Macklin, R. (2003) 'Dignity is a useless concept'. *British Medical Journal*, 327: 1419–29.

Maclean, A. (2001) 'Crossing the Rubicon on the Human Rights Ferry', *Modern Law Review*, 64: 784.

Magnusson, R.S. (2002) *Angels of Death*. London: Yale University Press.

Materstvedt, L.J. (2003) Palliative care on the 'slippery slope' towards euthanasia? *Palliative Medicine*, 17: 387–92.

Materstvedt, L.J., Clark, D., Ellershaw, J., Reidun, F., Gravaard, A.B., Mullerpbusch, C.H., Sales, J.P.I. and Rapin, C. (2003) Euthanasia and physician assisted suicide: a view from EAPC Ethics Task Force. *Palliative Medicine*, 17: 97–101.

Materstvedt, L.J. and Kaasa, S. (2000) Is terminal sedation active euthanasia? (Er terminal sedering aktiv dødshjelp?) *Tidsskr Nor Laegeforen*. (Journal of the Norwegian Medical Association). 10 June, 120(15): 1763–8.

May, C. (1992) Individual care? Power and subjectivity in therapeutic relationships. *Sociology*, 26: 589–602.

McNamara, B. (1998) A good enough death? in: A. Peterson and C. Waddell (eds) *Health Matters: A Sociology of Illness, Prevention and Care*. Sydney: Allen and Unwin, 169–84.

McNamara, B., Waddell, C. and Colvin, M. (1994) The institutionalization of the good death. *Social Science and Medicine*, 39(11): 1501–8.

Melzack, R. and Wall, P.D. (1988) *The Challenge of Pain*. London: Penguin.

Mill, J.S. (1859) On Liberty in: M. Warnock (ed.) 1977. *Utilitarianism*. Glasgow: Fontana.

Moody-Adams, M. (1999) The idea of moral progress. *Metaphilosophy*, 30(3): 168–85.

Mooney, G. (1994) *Key Issues in Health Economics*. New York, NY: Harvester Wheatsheaf.

Morris, D. (1997) Palliation: shielding the patient from the assault of symptoms. *Academy Update*, 7(3): 1–11.

Mount, B. (1997) The Royal Victoria Hospital Palliative Care Service: a Canadianexperience in: C. Saunders and R. Kastenbaum (eds) *Hospice Care on the International Scene*. New York, NY: Springer, 73–85.

Mulhall, S. and Swift, A. (1997) *Liberals and Communitarians*. 2nd edn. Oxford: Blackwell Publishers Ltd.

Murray, S.A., Kendall, M., Boyd, K. and Aziz, S. (2005) Illness trajectories and palliative care. *British Medical Journal*, 330: 1007–11.

Nagel, T. (1986) *The View From Nowhere*. New York, NY: Oxford University Press.

National Council for Hospices and Specialist Palliative Care Services (1995) *Specialist Palliative Care: A Statement of Definitions*. London: Occasional Paper 8.

National Council for Hospices and Specialist Palliative Care Services (1998) *Reaching Out: Specialist Palliative Care for Adults with Non-Malignant Diseases*. London: Occasional Paper 14.

National Health Service Confederation Report (2005) *Improving End-of-Life Care*, 12 November.

Nelson, J. L. (1992) Taking families seriously. *Hastings Centre Report*, 22(4): 6–12.

Nozick, R. (1984) *Philosophical Explanations*. Cambridge, MA: Harvard University Press.

Nussbaum, M. and Sen, A. (1993) *The Quality of Life*, Oxford: Clarendon Press.

Nunez-Olarte, J.M. and Gracia, D. (2001) Palliative care in Spain in: H. ten Have and R. Janssens (eds) *Palliative Care in Europe*. Amsterdam: IOS.

Oderberg, D.S. (2000a) *Applied Ethics: A Non-Consequentialist Approach*. Oxford: Blackwell.

Oderberg, D.S. (2000b) *Moral Theory: A Non-Consequentialist Approach*. Oxford: Blackwell.

Parfit, D. (1991) *Reasons and Persons*. 1st edn. reprint. Oxford: Clarendon Press.

Porta Sales, J. (2001) Sedation and terminal care. *European Journal of Palliative Care*, 8(3): 97–100.

Quill, T.E. and Byock, I.R. (2000) Responding to intractable suffering: the role of terminal sedation and voluntary refusal of food and fluids. *Annals of Internal Medicine*, 132: 408–14.

Quill. T.E., Coombs, L. B. and Nunn, S. (2000) Palliative Treatments of Last

Resort: choosing the least harmful alternative. *Annals of Internal Medicine*, 132: 488–93.

Randall, F. (2005) Letter to Select Committee: House of Lords (2005) *Select Committee on the Assisted Dying for the Terminally Ill Bill. Vol. II: Evidence.* London: The Stationery Office Limited.

Randall, F. and Downie, R.S. (1999) *Palliative Care Ethics: A Companion for all Specialties.* 2nd edn. Oxford: Oxford University Press.

Randall, F. and Downie, R.S. (2006) *The Philosophy of Palliative Care Critique and Reconstruction.* Oxford: Oxford University Press.

Raven, R.W. (1990) *The Theory and Practice of Oncology.* Carnforth: The Parthenon Publishing Group.

Rawls, J. (1993) *Political Liberalism.* New York, NY: Columbia University Press.

Rawls, J. (1971) *A Theory of Justice.* Oxford: Oxford University Press.

Raz, J. (1986) *The Morality of Freedom.* Oxford: Oxford University Press.

Robert, A.M. and Solomon, L. (2005) The challenge of human immunodeficiency virus: a model for palliative care. *Journal of Palliative Medicine*, 8(6): 1246–7.

Rousseau, P.C. (1996) Terminal sedation in the care of dying patients. *Arch Intern Med*, 156: 1785–6.

Royal College of Nursing Cancer Nursing Society (1996) *Guidelines for Good Practice in Cancer Nursing Education.* London.

Sacred Congregation for the Doctrine of the Faith (1980): *Declaration on Euthanasia.* Vatican City.

Sandman, L. (2005) *A Good Death: On the Value of Death and Dying.* Maidenhead: Open University Press.

Saunders, C. (1959) Care of the dying 1 – the problem of euthanasia. *Nursing Times.* 9 October, 960–1.

Saunders, C. (1960) Care of the dying. *Nursing Times Supplement.* London: Nursing Times reprint.

Saunders, C. (1962) Working at St Joseph's Hospice, Hackney. *Annual Report of St. Vincent's Dublin*, 37–39.

Saunders, C. (1964) The care of the dying – how we can help? *Medical News.* 21 February, 7.

Saunders, C. (1965) The last stages of life. *American Journal of Nursing*, 65: 70–5.

Saunders, C. (1966) The management of terminal illness. *British Journal of Hospital Medicine.* December, 225–8.

Saunders, C. (1967) The care of the dying. *Gerontologica Clinica*, 9: 385–90.

Saunders, C. (1969) The moment of truth: care of the dying person in: L. Pearson (ed.) *Death and Dying: Current Issues in the Treatment of the Dying Person.* Cleveland OH: The Press of Case Western Reserve University, 49–78.

Saunders, C. (1972) The care of the dying patient and his family. *Contact.* Suppl. 38 Summer, 12–28.

Saunders, C. (1973) A place to die. *Crux*, 11(3): 24–7.

Saunders, C. (1976) Care of the dying – the problem of euthanasia (2) *Nursing Times*, (72)27: 1049–52.

Saunders, C. (1986) The modern hospice in: F. Wald (ed.) *In quest of the Spiritual Component of Care for the Terminally Ill.* Yale, CT: Yale University School of Nursing.

Saunders, C. (1987a) I was sick and you visited me. *Christian Nurse International*

3(4): 4–5.

Saunders, C. (1987b) What's in a name? *Palliative Medicine*, 1: 57–61.

Saunders, C. (1993) Foreword in: D. Doyle, G.W.C. Hanks and N. MacDonald, (eds) *Oxford textbook of palliative medicine*. Oxford: Oxford University Press, v-viii.

Saunders, C. (1994/95) Past, present and future hospice and palliative care. *History of Nursing Journal*, 5: 43–5.

Saunders, C. (1995) In Britain: fewer conflicts of conscience. *Hastings Centre Report*. May-June, 25(3) 44–5.

Saunders, C. (1996) Into the valley of the shadow of death: a personal therapeutic journey. *British Medical Journal*, 313(13): 1599–1601.

Saunders, C. (2003) *Watch with me*. Sheffield: Mortal Press.

Saunders, C. (2005) Foreword in: D. Doyle, G. Hanks, N. Cherny, K. Calman (eds) *Oxford Textbook of Palliative Medicine*. 3rd edn. Oxford: Oxford University Press.

Savulescu, J. (1997) Liberal rationalism and medical decision-making. *Bioethics*, 11(2): 115–29.

Schneiderman, L.J. (1991) Is it morally justifiable not to sedate this patient before ventilator removal? *The Journal of Clinical Ethics*, 2: 129–30.

Seale, C. (1989) What happens in hospices: a review of the literature. *Social Science and Medicine*, 28(6): 551–9.

Seale, C. (1991) Death from cancer and other causes: the relevance of the hospice approach. *Palliative Medicine*, 5(1): 12–9.

Seale, C. (1995) Heroic Death. *Sociology*, 29(4): 597–613.

Seale, C. and Cartwright, A. (1994) *The Year Before Death*. Avebury: Aldershot.

Seymour, J.E. (2001) *Critical Moments: Death and Dying in Intensive Care*. Buckingham: Open University Press.

Singer, P. (1994) *Rethinking Life and Death*. Oxford: Oxford University Press.

Singer, P. (1995) *Practical Ethics*. 2nd Edn. Cambridge: Cambridge University Press.

Slevin, M.L., Stubbs, L., Plant, H.J., Downer, S.M., Armes, P.J., Wilson, P. and Gregory, W.M. (1990) Attitudes to Chemotherapy: comparing views of cancer patients with those of doctors, nurses, and general public. *British Medical Journal*, 300: 1458–60.

Smith, A. (1759) *A Theory of Moral Sentiments*. Indianapolis, in: Liberty Classics 1976.

Standing Medical Advisory Committee/Standing Nursing and Midwifery Advisory Committee (SMAC/SNMAC) (1992) *The Principles and Provision of Palliative Care*. London: HMSO.

Stauch, M. (2002) Comment on Re B. (Adult refusal of medical treatment) [2002] 2 All England Reports 449. *Journal of Medical Ethics*, 28: 232–3.

Steinbock, B. (1992) *Life Before Birth: The Moral and Legal Status of Embryos and Foetuses*. New York, NY: Oxford University Press.

Swarte, N.B., van der Lee, M.L., van der Bom, J.G., van den Bout, J. and Heintz, A.P.M. (2003) Effects of euthanasia on the bereaved family and friends: A cross sectional study. *British Medical Journal*, 327: 189–94.

Tännsjö, T. (2000) Terminal sedation: A possible compromise in the euthanasia debate? *Bulletin of Medical Ethics*. November 13–22.

Tännsjö, T. (2002) *Understanding Ethics: An Introduction to Moral Theory.* Edinburgh: Edinburgh University Press.

Tännsjö, T. (ed.) (2004) *Terminal Sedation.* Dordrecht: Kluwer Academic Press.

Taylor, C. (1985) *Philosophy and the Human Sciences.* Cambridge: Cambridge University Press.

Taylor, C. (1990) *Sources of the Self.* Cambridge, MA: Cambridge University Press.

Taylor, R.M. and Lantos, J.D. (1995) *The Politics of Medical Futility.* Issues in Law and Medicine 3.

ten Have, H. and Clark, D. (eds) *The Ethics of Palliative Care: European Perspectives.* Buckingham: Open University Press.

Thomas, K. (2003) *Caring for the Dying at Home: Companions on the Journey.* Oxford: Radcliffe Medical Press.

Thomas, L. (2000) Moral Psychology in: H. LaFollette (ed.) *The Blackwell Guide to Ethical Theory.* Oxford: Blackwell, 149–62.

Thorpe, G. (1993) Enabling more dying people to remain at home. *British Medical Journal*, 307: 915–8.

Tiffany, R. (1990) A core curriculum for a course in palliative nursing care. *Palliative Medicine*, 4: 261–2.

Tobias, J.S. (1997) BMJ's present policy: (sometimes approving research in which patients have not given fully informed consent) is wholly correct. *British Medical Journal*, 314: 1111–4.

Troug, D., Arnold, K.H. and Rockoff, M.A. (1991) Sedation before ventilator removal: Medical and Ethical considerations. *The Journal of Clinical Ethics*, 2: 127.

Twycross, R. (1990) *Therapeutics in Terminal Cancer.* London: Churchill Livingstone.

Twycross, R. and Lack, S. (1993) *Oral Morphine in Advanced Cancer.* Revised 2nd edn. England: Beaconsfield Publishers Limited.

Veatch, R. M. (1995) Abandoning informed consent. *Hastings Centre Report*, 25(2): 5–12.

Ventafridda, B., Ripamonti, C., DeConn, F., Tamburini, F. and Cassileth, B.R. (1990) Symptom prevalence and control during cancer patient's last days of life. *Journal of Palliative Care*, 6(3): 7–11.

Waldron, J. (1987) The theoretical foundations of liberalism. *Philosophical Quarterly*, 37(147): 127–50.

Walter, T. (1991) Modern Death: Taboo or not taboo? *Sociology*, 25(2): 293–310.

Walter, T. (1997a) The ideology and organization of spiritual care: three approaches. *Palliative Medicine*, 11: 21–30.

Walter, T. (1997b) *The Eclipse of Eternity: A Sociology of the Afterlife.* Basingstoke: Macmillan.

Walter, T. (2003) Historical and cultural variants on the good death. *British Medical Journal*, 327: 218–20.

Walters, G. (2004) Is there such a thing as a good death? *Palliative Medicine*, 5(1): 404–8.

Wanzer, S.H., Federman, D.D. and Adelstein, S.J. (1989) The physician's responsibility toward hopelessly ill patients: a second look. *New England Journal of Medicine*, 120: 844–9.

Warnock, M. (1983) In vitro fertilisation: The ethical issues (II). *The Philosophical*

Quarterly, 132: 238–2497.

Weijer, C. (2000) 'Family duty is more important than rights'. *British Medical Journal*, 321(9): 1466.

Wilkes, E. (1993) Introduction in: D. Clark (ed.) *The Future For Palliative Care*. Buckingham: Open University Press.

Williams, R. (1990) *The Protestant Legacy: Attitudes to Death And Illness Among Older Aberdonians*. Oxford: Clarendon Press.

Wittgenstein, L. (1958) *Philosophical Investigations*. Trans. G.E.M. Anscombe. Oxford: Basil Blackwell.

Woods, S. (1998) 'Holism' in: S.D. Edwards (ed.) *The Philosophy of Nursing*. London: Macmillan, 67–88.

Woods, S. (2000) Persons and personal identity. *Nursing Philosophy*, 1(2): 169–72.

Woods, S. (2001) The contribution of nursing to the development of palliative care in: H. ten Have and R. Janssens (eds) *Palliative Care in Europe*. Amsterdam: IOS, 133–42.

Woods, S. (2004a) Terminal sedation: a nursing perspective in: T. Tännsjö (ed.) *Terminal Sedation*. Dordrecht: Kluwer Academic Press.

Woods, S. (2004b) Is terminal sedation compatible with good nursing care at the end of life? *International Journal of Palliative Nursing*, 10(5): 244–7.

Woods, S. (2005a) Respect for persons: autonomy and palliative care. *Medicine HealthCare and Philosophy*, 8: 243–53.

Woods, S. (2005b) Moral Progress in: M. Hayry and T. Takala (eds.) *Ethics and Social Realism*. New York, NY: Rodopi.

Woods, S. (2006) Saving the anthropomorphic person in: S. Holm, T. Takala and M. Hayry (eds) *Life of Value – John Harris, His Arguments and His Critics*, (forthcoming). New York, NY: Rodopi.

Woods, S., Beaver, K. and Luker, K. (2000) User's views of palliative care services: ethical implications. *Nursing Ethics*, 7(4): 314–26.

Woods, S. and Elstein, M. (2002) Care home ethics in: J. Humber and R. Almedar (eds.) *Care of the Aged*. Biomedical Ethics Series: Humana Press. 103–28.

Woods, S., Webb, P. and Clark, D. (2001) Palliative care in the United Kingdom in: H. ten Have and R. Janssens (eds) *Palliative Care in Europe*. Amsterdam: IOS, 85–98.

World Health Organisation (1990) *Cancer Pain Relief and Palliative Care*. Technical report series 804. Geneva: WHO.

World Health Organisation (2002) *Cancer Pain Relief in Palliative Care*. Technical Report Series. Geneva: WHO.

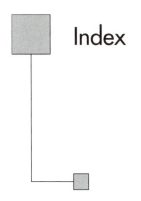

Index